HOW DIETS MAKE US FAT

SHAHROO IZADI

HOW DIETS MAKE US FAT

The book the diet industry doesn't want you to read

LEAP

First published in the UK in 2025 by LEAP
An imprint of Bonnier Books UK
5th Floor, HYLO, 105 Bunhill Row,
London, EC1Y 8LZ

Copyright © Roocovery Limited, 2025

All rights reserved.

No part of this publication may be reproduced, stored or transmitted in any form or by any means, electronic, mechanical, photocopying or otherwise, without the prior written permission of the publisher.

The right of Shahroo Izadi to be identified as Author of this work has been asserted by her in accordance with the Copyright, Designs and Patents Act, 1988.

A CIP catalogue record for this book is available from the British Library.

Hardback ISBN: 978-1-78512-277-4
Trade Paperback ISBN: 978-1-78512-431-0

Also available as an ebook and an audiobook

1 3 5 7 9 10 8 6 4 2

Design and Typeset by Envy Design Ltd
Printed and bound by CPI Group (UK) Ltd, Croydon CR0 4YY

Every reasonable effort has been made to trace copyright holders of material reproduced in this book, but if any have been inadvertently overlooked the publishers would be glad to hear from them.

The authorised representative in the EEA is
Bonnier Books UK (Ireland) Limited.
Registered office address:
Block B, The Crescent Building
Northwood, Santry
Dublin 9, D09 C6X8, Ireland
compliance@bonnierbooks.ie

www.bonnierbooks.co.uk

To Ferri

Contents

Introduction	1
1: How I Know	11
2: A New Paradigm	31

PART 1: What Happens When You Diet — 39

3: How You Know	40
4: The Myth of the Addictive Personality	45
5: The Information Prison	59
6: When Emotional Eating Stops Feeling Like Comfort	67
7: When Your Food Landscape Shrinks	79
8: The Self-Sabotage Trap	89
9: The Knowledge-Action Gap	99
10: Joining the Dots	109

PART 2: The Bigger Picture — 119

11: Shame: The Invisible Accelerant — 120
12: Why Some People Get Trapped Faster — 131
13: The Abusive Relationship with Diet Culture — 143
14: Why Nothing Else Has Worked — 155
15: A Different Kind of Recovery — 165

PART 3: The Way Out — 173

16: The Beginning of Behavioral Change — 174
17: The Power Recovery Framework — 179
18: Step 1 – Power Assessment — 189
19: Step 2 – Creating Your Baseline — 205
20: Step 3 – The Bridge Days — 219
21: Step 4 – Building Your Flight Record — 227
22: Step 5 – Reclaiming Your Hands — 245
23: Step 6 – Reclaiming Forbidden Territory — 253
24: Step 7 – Changing Your Internal Script — 265
25: Step 8 – Emotional Regulation Without Food — 281
26: Step 9 – Real-Life Application — 287
27: Step 10 – Long-Term Maintenance and Your Comprehensive Toolkit — 293

References — 308

Introduction

Let me take a wild guess . . . You already know that diets screw people over. That's why you're reading this book.

After years of trying so hard to lose weight, your relationship with food is still chaotic. Do you even remember a time when you could just eat a meal without over-thinking it? When you didn't feel like you were one 'bad food choice' away from disaster? When you actually knew what hunger felt like, instead of constantly second-guessing your body? There's something deeper happening here – a frustrating paradox where the harder you chase thinness, the further away it seems to drift.

By now your diet CV would impress even the most hardcore weight-loss gurus. WeightWatchers? Check. Keto? Been there. Intermittent fasting? Atkins? Those chalky meal replacement shakes? Done, done and unfortunately done. You could seriously teach a masterclass in macronutrients at this point.

But here's the wildest part – each diet attempt becomes harder to sustain. The control periods get shorter. The rebounds get more intense. Never eating again feels more achievable than eating flexibly – whatever that means anymore. Alternatively, drinking three bland shakes a day feels simpler than figuring out regular meals.

And those magical moments when you were actually happy with your weight? They've been painfully brief because maintaining your target weight feels impossible.

I'm here to tell you that you're not possessed, stupid or uniquely incapable of eating like a 'normal person'. Instead, you've been trying to win a game that's rigged against you in every possible way – and the longer it goes on, the more you convince yourself you can crack it if only you try harder, or if you just want thinness *enough*.

But here's what nobody wants to admit: diet culture doesn't just fail to help you lose weight and keep weight off permanently. It actively damages your relationship with food, your body, and your sense of personal power in ways that make weight management progressively more difficult.

And you're not alone. I, like you and millions of others, have also been brainwashed – gaslit – into thinking that without a diet to follow, I will 'sabotage' myself, spiral into inevitable chaos and end up bigger than I was when I began my latest diet.

I turned that belief into a self-fulfilling prophecy without even realising it, until it was easier to eat nothing at all than to 'eat everything in moderation'. (I hate that saying, and I imagine you do too.)

HOW DIETS MAKE US FAT

The fact is, what you've been experiencing isn't happening in a vacuum. We are living in unprecedented times. We are bombarded with more weight-loss products, food rules, and conflicting health information than any other generation in human history. Social media feeds us a constant stream of before-and-after photos, transformation stories, and impossible body standards. Every grocery store aisle, every restaurant menu, every social gathering has become a minefield of choices that feel morally loaded.

We also have access to more weight-loss options and diet advice than ever before – intermittent fasting, plant-based, carnivore, macro counting, intuitive eating, medical weight loss, surgical interventions. Yet obesity rates keep climbing. The more solutions become available, the more powerless, confused and 'broken' people feel around food.

What I'll Show You

In Part 1 of this book, I'm going to detail your likely current behaviors – the ones you're blaming yourself for right now – and walk you through what is actually happening to your mind and body as a result of dieting, and how it's left you feeling powerless.

My guess is that you've never changed the way you eat if not to lose weight. Maybe you decided to become vegan or go gluten free for health reasons at some point, but you were probably still hoping that the scales would drop as a result.

Maybe eating 'sensibly' feels impossible for you, and you can relate to an alcoholic who finds it easier not to drink than to have just one; perhaps you wish you didn't have to eat at all.

Maybe you're always going to extremes – when you're 'good' with food, you're really good. When you're 'bad', you're really bad. You can't seem to find that middle ground which other people apparently navigate so easily.

Maybe you've noticed that certain foods – especially processed foods – seem to have a greater hold over you than other people. You can't just have one biscuit or one handful of crisps. It's all-or-nothing, and 'all' usually wins.

Maybe you're someone who succeeds at everything else in life. You can manage complex projects, make difficult decisions, and solve problems that stump other people – but you just can't figure out how to eat 'normally'.

I want to show you the truth: diet culture has trained you to distrust your own instincts, override your body's signals, and see natural, necessary human responses to restriction as personal failures. Every diet you've ever tried has reinforced the message that your natural hunger, your food preferences, and your body's needs are wrong and must be controlled.

You didn't develop these patterns because you're weak or broken. You developed them because you've been subjected to a system that benefits from eliciting these responses while convincing you that you are the one to blame.

HOW DIETS MAKE US FAT

The Invisible Accelerator

Then there's the hidden component that turbocharges this entire problem into something that feels completely unmanageable: shame.

Every time you 'fail' at a diet, you don't just feel disappointed about not losing weight. You feel ashamed of yourself. This shame is so unbearable that your brain looks for immediate relief – and food provides that relief. So you eat more, which generates more shame, which makes you eat even more. You're not just eating the biscuit – you're eating to numb the pain of feeling like someone who can't resist a biscuit.

And the cruelest part of the trap? The diet industry profits from your shame. It needs you to feel broken, powerless, and dependent on its solutions. If you truly believed you could trust yourself around food, you'd stop buying diet products, joining weight-loss programmes, and listening to the endless stream of conflicting advice that keeps the industry profitable.

But your shame *isn't* a flaw – as I'll show you in Part 2, it's the predictable result of being told repeatedly that your most basic human needs are moral failings. You feel guilty for being hungry. You feel weak for wanting foods that taste good. You feel broken for having a body that responds to restriction with increased desire for food.

The longer this goes on, the more you neglect, abuse and confuse yourself because you've normalized feeling neglected, abused and confused. You become your own worst critic, your harshest judge, your most relentless attacker. You internalize the voice that tells you your struggles are your fault, that your hunger is wrong, that your body is the enemy, thereby creating the exact emotional conditions that make you want to eat more. Shame doesn't prevent powerless overeating – it drives it.

Why You Might be Extra Vulnerable

There are also some people for whom conventional diet approaches are genuinely harder to follow. If you have Attention Deficit Hyperactivity Disorder (ADHD), for example, your brain craves immediate reward and novelty – but sustainable eating requires delayed gratification and routine. Extreme dieting exploits this vulnerability by offering you the immediate high of restriction and the rebellion of bingeing, both of which trigger your reward system more intensely than they would in other brains.

Likewise, if you're naturally a perfectionist, your brain interprets any deviation as complete failure – yet long-term behavior change requires you to accept imperfect progress. Diet culture feeds your all-or-nothing thinking while setting up conditions that make perfection impossible to maintain.

If you learned early that your worth was tied to your appearance, every food choice feels like a moral emergency rather than a simple decision. If you've experienced trauma, stress, or a difficult childhood, food may have become your primary source of comfort and control.

But you're not failing at simple instructions – you're trying to follow instructions that weren't designed for the way your brain uniquely works, or the way any brain works. This is why I've dedicated a whole chapter to readers who are neurodivergent or who have experienced trauma and are very familiar with a sense of failure, shame and all-or-nothing thinking when it comes to food. Understanding your specific vulnerabilities isn't about making excuses – it's about embracing approaches that work *with* your brain rather than against it.

What I Won't Waste Your Time With

You already know that diets don't work for sustainable weight loss. You know this because you've tried them. Multiple times. You've lost weight and gained it back, often ending up heavier than when you started.

You also suspect that weight-loss drugs, while they can be effective tools, won't address the underlying psychological patterns that have created your struggles with food. Many people using these medications still feel anxious and out of control around food – they're just not as physically hungry. And they have no idea how they're ever going to come off them.

Nor am I going to encourage you to follow a diet disguised as 'lifestyle change'. I'm not going to tell you to eat mindfully, listen to your body, or be intuitive. For someone whose relationship with food has been systematically damaged, those approaches create more stress, not less.

I'm not going to pretend that 'body positivity' works when you're bigger than you want to be, as a direct result of abuse and neglect when it comes to powerless choices towards your body; or that 'food freedom' and 'winging it' will work for someone whose brain naturally operates in extreme ways, either. If, like me, you're someone who finds it impossible to have just one of anything, simply removing all structure doesn't create balance – it creates chaos. For us, 'more is more'; and sensible plans don't only backfire, the very idea of them bores the hell out of us.

And I'm never going to patronize you with the 'restriction is unhealthy' line, when I know you know that, and I know that restriction is the closest you think you can get to putting the brakes on rapid weight gain and quietening your constant internal chatter around food.

What I Will Do

In the final part of this book, I'm going to reveal a process that will teach you, step by step, how to reclaim your power over food. This process will offer you a long-term solution that will finally free you from the diet treadmill that's been failing you.

It's a framework for undoing the damage that made you believe you couldn't trust yourself in the first place. This approach draws on methods used in the clinical addiction recovery field, acknowledging that sustainable change only happens through learning and skill-building. Addiction recovery doesn't expect people to be perfect from day one. It expects setbacks, builds in support for difficult moments, and treats every slip as information rather than failure.

HOW DIETS MAKE US FAT

Most importantly, addiction recovery understands that change happens choice by choice, and shame is the enemy of change. It actively works to reduce shame because it knows that shame creates the exact conditions that make compulsive behavior more likely. This is the opposite of diet culture, which uses shame as its primary motivational tool.

If you've genuinely collected evidence that you can't eat one slice of toast, one piece of chocolate, or go on one holiday without spiralling out of control, no one should be trying to convince you otherwise. So I don't expect you to believe right now that you can lose weight and keep it off. I don't expect you to believe that you can control yourself to make any choice you like, or that eating healthily or in a calm way will ever be possible. I don't need you to believe in your ability to do something you've proven you can't do for a long time.

But I *do* need you to believe in just one thing: mastery. I need you to believe that if you practice any choices using the tools in a row (helped by the tool I'm going to teach you), they *will* become easier.

This time around, the plan isn't going to be informed by what is physically 'healthy'. You don't need that. Instead, I will train you to stop doing the things that you know are mentally unhealthy for you. You know as well as I do that losing weight isn't the problem – gaining it back is. So you need to be mentally fit enough to behave like a calm, mature, wise person when it comes to what you eat – and in all your choices.

You don't need to learn how to eat. You just need to learn to stop relinquishing your power to a diet industry that has massively short-changed you and persuaded you that you need it, even though it's the very reason you're stuck.

If you join me on this journey, you'll break free from that programming while finally achieving the weight-loss results you deserve. You'll come to realize that your perceived powerlessness over food was an illusion created by a system that was profiting from your struggle. This method gives you back what was always yours: the ability to trust yourself completely around food, to eat in a way that serves you, and to prove to yourself that you were never broken.

Think of this book as a good friend who has already broken free – someone who knows that, right now, you don't believe you can do it. Yet they will walk you through it anyway because they know the steps you need to take.

Trust this friend to guide you back to yourself – and never doubt your own abilities again.

Chapter 1

How I Know: My Own Failed Dieting Story

I know your story because I've been the same obsessive dieter who could recite calorie counts in my sleep. I've been the secret binger hiding wrappers at the bottom of the bin. I've been the Monday morning warrior swearing: 'This time is different!' while my body screamed otherwise. In fact, throughout most of my childhood, I was diet culture's perfect student.

From the age of around ten, I became concerned about the increasing size of my body. Growing up, I had not experienced the world as a slim person. I was really quite fat by most countries' standards, let alone the UK and the USA where I spent my childhood. Looking back, I realize I internalized the clear message that thin is good and fat is bad. This pervasive message, and the omnipresent influence of diet culture, took root early, instilling in me a subconscious belief. It was simply a 'fact' absorbed from the world I was born into.

I came to understand that being thin was not only desirable but essential – the only state that promised success, happiness and popularity. And, in the 1990s, it wasn't difficult to find evidence that reinforced this belief. Television programmes often portrayed bigger women as laughable for wanting boyfriends, or as people who had to compensate for their size with funny personalities and a lack of boundaries: someone like Monica from the TV sitcom *Friends* (portrayed by slim actor Courteney Cox in a fat suit). In the 1990s, 'Nothing tastes as good as skinny feels' became diet culture's rallying cry. It was a time when you could visit a friend's house and their mother would have no problem saying that you might want to think about losing a few pounds (and it was considered polite to thank her for her helpful advice).

I had connected food to weight, and weight to self-worth, for as long as I could remember. Before I knew there was potassium in a banana, or even what potassium was, I knew from a magazine I found at the hairdresser's that bananas are high in sugar and therefore unhelpful for losing weight. Every Monday represented a new start, the chance of a transformation, a final attempt to achieve the thinness I longed for.

The Shame Begins

My first memory of shame around food was when I was around 11. I took two blueberry cereal bars from my uncle's house, where I'd been staying for the summer holiday,

HOW DIETS MAKE US FAT

and I stashed them behind a cushion so that I could eat them later.

At this point, I was already very overweight compared to other children my age and since I was fortunate enough that food scarcity wasn't a problem, I'd probably realized that cereal bars were 'bad' – not for all kids, but for kids like me. And not because cereal bars were unhealthy, either. In fact, these products were often advertised as health foods, but I knew somehow that they weren't okay for me.

By this point, kids were making fun of me at school; the GP was prescribing diets even if I went in for a cold, and everyone who loved me was, of course, trying to support me by encouraging me not to eat too much. After all, they knew the harsh reality: life is harder if you're fat. When it came to bedtime – the time for me to be alone with my snacks – my uncle came to make the sofa bed up for me. When he lifted the cushions and the cereal bars fell out, I was horrified. I felt so guilty and ashamed. I knew I'd been caught.

Even at that young age, I knew that I should feel bad if I'd done something that would make everyone else unhappy with me – something I knew people 'like me' shouldn't do. My uncle made a joke and took the bars away, and I remember lying in bed that night, asking myself for the first time: *Why do I have to be different? Why is so much wrong with me? Why is my body bad?*

I became hyper-aware of what other children could eat freely while I could not. I began wanting to go over to my friends' houses, especially those whose parents allowed 'naughty' foods that I wasn't allowed at home. I didn't really understand what I was doing wrong. And today, it's heartbreaking for me to reflect on the fact that I immediately took responsibility for the size of my body at an age when I wasn't required to take responsibility for anything else.

The Feast and Famine Cycle Begins

It started predictably enough: I was just a kid trying to get her hands on the delicious foods that seemed to have suddenly disappeared from my home, and from my plate in other people's houses. Then, as a teenager, I began taking appetite suppressants and white-knuckling through absurd restrictive diets. Eventually, a pattern emerged: giving in when a diet of boiled eggs and cabbage soup became unbearable, or when the weight wasn't dropping off quickly enough to justify the hunger and deprivation.

In those moments, I started eating foods that I'd barely thought about before, in larger and larger quantities and very quickly too. Falling off the wagon of restrictive dieting made me realize how exhilarating, euphoric, even numbing, large quantities of fatty, sugary foods could be. Little did I know, this cycle was laying the foundations for me to develop an emotional dependence on food.

Every week, I would start a new diet, if you could even call it that. Usually it was something as ridiculous as eating only tomatoes one day and only meat another day. Or, if I was really disappointed with myself because someone had made a comment about my weight, I would get even more restrictive. Sometimes I would decide to live only on celery for as long as possible. Naturally, because I was overweight, I was applauded for the effect these choices had on my body. Suddenly, I was looking a lot thinner.

Of course, these periods of living off cucumber and compliments never lasted long. Over time, my starvation stints got shorter and shorter, while the periods of rebellion and abandon around food grew longer and more intense. Even so, this didn't register as a problem, since I never over-ate without believing with every fibre of my being that it was the last time it would happen. In fact, the only way I could justify each period of being 'bad' – when I was knowingly on a mission to eat as much unhealthy food as possible – was by convincing myself it would be my last hurrah.

I kept taking two hopeful steps forwards, then five shameful steps back. I would starve myself from Monday until Thursday and only manage to lose a fraction of the weight I had gained between Friday and Sunday the previous week. Every Monday morning, I would wake up more disappointed with myself. I was absolutely convinced that my desperation to be thin, compounded by my shame at allowing myself to get so fat, would be enough to keep me on track. Yet every Monday morning, I woke up a little further from my goal, for reasons I didn't even understand: diminished self-belief, binge-induced weight gain, and withdrawal symptoms after my Sunday night 'final binge', which always brought acid reflux, lethargy, and intense sugar cravings.

The University Years: When Everything Intensified

By the time I arrived at university to study psychology, I was constantly either rapidly gaining or losing weight. I'd never established an enjoyable, healthy, varied, routine and sensible way of eating. I had absolutely no interest in my mental or physical health. This wasn't helped by the fact that I was continually reminded that being overweight was the most physically repulsive thing you could possibly be. Not only did I internalize the belief that my body wasn't worth taking care of while I was fat, but I also reinforced it – a lot! If I wasn't thin, or on the way to being thin, I wasn't engaging in any self-care at all. No water to drink, no make-up, no music. That stuff's for thin people!

At this point, you might be wondering why I kept going back for more. Why, if diets clearly weren't making me slimmer, did I keep persevering with them? The truth is, I didn't know any other route to achieve the holy grail of weight loss and, technically, diets weren't to blame – I was. I never connected my inability to stop overeating with anything other than greed and weakness.

What was I supposed to think? Was I meant to stop trying to lose weight when I was at my heaviest, when it felt like the most important thing in the world? To go back to what? Since I was stuck in a 'feast or famine' mindset, I believed the brief periods of restriction were the only times I wasn't getting rapidly heavier. As far as I was concerned, diets had delivered, but I hadn't. Diets could be trusted, but

I couldn't be. Diets told me what to eat and what not to eat to lose weight quickly. If I could just stop being so weak, lazy and greedy, and stick to the rules forever, everything would be sorted!

Plus, the effectiveness of diets couldn't be denied. As long as I did exactly what the diet prescribed, as long as I didn't cheat next time, didn't socialize next time, and never stopped tracking every morsel I ate, the diet would do its job. Then if I decided to stop following the rules, if I let myself and the diet down, if I didn't keep my side of the bargain – well, that was on me.

It was very similar to the trajectory of substance abuse. The less effective the dietary restriction became, the more I chased some return on my investment. By this point, I had nothing to lose and nowhere to go but back to the diet cult I was addicted to, with a promise that, this time, I was desperate enough to do better. And the more weight I gained, the more dependent I became on the cult to save me from myself. By now, I was 10 years into spending every single day comparing my body to other people's. I kept wondering why I was bigger than them, dreaded getting dressed up to go out, and ultimately, by the age of 21, I weighed 120kg. I was both the fattest person and the most compulsive dieter around.

The Dark Realities of Living Large

Looking back, I can't believe the extent of my disgust with myself and my body. My binges would make my skin itch because I developed stretch marks. I always gained weight in the lead-up to an event, even if I was trying to lose it. Little did I know that every diet, every 'fat camp', every laxative, was a false economy that offered diminishing returns.

I realize now that food was the bane of my life. I was always either terrified of eating or not eating. It controlled every aspect of my existence – so much so that during my second year of university, I ramped things up and had gastric-band surgery. This was one defeat I admitted to myself, but not to anyone else because I did it in secret. That alone is testament to how much shame I carried. I am normally not only an over-sharer but a person who is terrified by the thought of needles and operations.

Initially after the surgery I was told I'd be able to eat as much as I had done before. This was because the band had been installed around my upper stomach and it was loose enough so that I wouldn't feel it. Once I'd recovered, I could return to the clinic to get it tightened, depending on my needs. The looser I asked for it to stay, the more I could eat. The tighter I had it made, the less I'd be able to eat.

At first, in that pre-tightening post-op stage, I ate almost nothing. Then, predictably, before my first band-tightening appointment, I went back to eating everything 'one last time'. I really went for it. *Why wouldn't I?* After all, this time I didn't need to rely on myself to get thin. I could rely on the band from now on. So, of course, this *was* going to be the last, last time!

During that first follow-up consultation, I was reminded of how badly I wanted – how badly I needed – to be thin at any cost. The surgeon tightened the band by inserting a large needle into my abdomen that sent liquid into the band, filling it up so it tightened around my stomach. That way, if I ate too much, I simply wouldn't be able to swallow it. I'd have to take the food out of my mouth, break it into smaller pieces, and chew it longer. To make matters worse, because of what the band does to your gag reflex, when food did manage to go down, it was easy to bring it back up. The bulimia I'd never succeeded in inducing before was suddenly available.

I had no interest in learning how to eat sensibly or live long-term with the band. As far as I was concerned, it was the next best thing to wiring my jaw shut. I was losing weight quickly, so I kept asking the surgeon to tighten the band as much as possible. Essentially I was using it to starve myself.

At one stage, the gastric band enabled me to lose so much weight that, for the first time in my life, I wasn't a fat person. I wasn't even a slim person. I was a very, very slim person. And my whole world changed. When I lost a lot of weight, it confirmed what I already knew. The world does treat you differently. I was constantly applauded: people assumed all sorts of unrelated aspects of my life must be going well, and everyone wanted to know what my secret was. But I couldn't tell them. I was terrified that anyone would discover I'd taken the 'easy way out'.

Before long, I was in and out of the clinic for around a year, asking for extreme loosening or tightening and playing out my old pattern even more extremely. For 18 months I cycled between extreme tightening and loosening, living my restriction-rebellion pattern at its most extreme. Each tightening brought weight loss and control. Each loosening brought rebellion and regain. After wild fluctuations, I demanded it be tightened one final time. Too tight. Something ruptured – not just physically. I ended up back in surgery. The surgeon explained he'd had to remove it. The band had caused complications requiring removal. I cried with relief. I wanted my own body back.

For the first time I allowed myself to admit how horrible it had been to be governed by something that felt so alien and that had normalized not only hunger but also physical pain. Thankfully, my unexpected but clear response to the band being removed made me realize I had hit rock bottom. It was time for therapy, a practice I went on to keep as a fixture in my life for stints (ranging from three to twelve months) over the following decade.

Therapy: The Beginning of Real Change

I remember my first therapy session clearly. As soon as I sat down, I made it clear to my counsellor that I wasn't ready to get on board with loving my body at any size. I was just about ready to believe that a few conversations about why I ate so much might help me stick to a diet long enough to be thin. As I was still in my twenties, I thought I was young enough to turn things around – to live the rest of my life as a thin person.

But then something strange happened. As I got to know my therapist, things began to change. I rarely, if ever, missed a therapy session. I liked her. She didn't control the conversation. Nor did she let me get away with much. When I presented information as fact when it was only my opinion, she challenged me and taught me to challenge myself. Whenever I told her a story in a way that conveniently painted me in a better light than I deserved, she called me out on it. She was also unshockable so I kept revealing more and more, waiting for her to judge me or to display an emotion other than her usual neutral response.

Pretty soon she passed whatever criteria I subconsciously had for a therapist, and so I went all in. I told her everything. I told her the worst things I said to myself, and the less-than-kind thoughts I had about other people. I came to trust this woman and enjoyed how honest I could be; so much so that I looked forward to coming clean to her about the lies I had told the week before. This honesty was a revolutionary experience for someone who had spent years hiding her eating, lying about her weight, and pretending to be someone she wasn't. For the first time, I was completely honest about my struggles without being met by judgment, advice, or attempts to 'fix me'.

Through therapy, I realized that my life had become a never-ending preparation for thinness, during which I gained weight and then planned again for my better life. The brief periods when I was thin were just a waiting room for failure. Ironically, the process of unpacking painful stories from my past allowed me to take a much less personal view of the powerless state I was in. It enabled me to go from thinking: *How did I let this happen?* To: *There's literally no other way this could have gone.* It helped me think about my problem objectively and have compassion for myself, the way I would for any human being.

Then, the penny finally dropped. A few months into our sessions, my therapist asked how I would feel if I never got thin. I was furious. *She doesn't get me at all!* I thought. *How could she even suggest I might spend my whole life looking like this?* I believed every aspect of my life would be worse. There would be nothing to look forward to, and the best things in life would never be available to me.

The question was also interesting because my therapist was visibly overweight herself, and she made a point of telling me she had no problem with this during our sessions. In the early days of therapy, when she said this, I thought, *Rubbish! We're living in the same world.* I couldn't fathom anyone accepting – let alone preferring – their body at a larger size.

This is how deeply ingrained my thinking was. Being fat was bad; and it wasn't just me who I thought was bad; it was everyone. I believed anyone who was overweight would be happier if they weren't, even though I had no idea of what they were going through in their lives. This was also despite the fact that when I had been thinner, I hadn't necessarily been happier. In fact, I was often particularly anxious when I managed to become really slim – because I was scared it wouldn't last.

After that session, where I was forced to consider what life might be like if I lived as a fat person (a nightmare scenario!), I decided to go for a walk to clear my head. As I strolled across London Bridge, mentally rehearsing the 'you don't get me' speech planned to give my therapist in our next session, I became more aware of other overweight people.

HOW DIETS MAKE US FAT

I realized that, while I believed they'd be happier and probably healthier if they weren't so fat, I didn't think they deserved to neglect their mental and physical health completely or only drink water when they'd earned it by being thin. They didn't deserve to feel silly when they made an effort to get their hair done. They didn't need to feel thin to enjoy a holiday.

It dawned on me that I had turned the idea of 'fat means worthless' into a self-fulfilling prophecy. Over the years, as I'd gained more weight and become more ashamed of it, the weight had reinforced my belief that my faulty, weak, betraying body wasn't worth taking care of. This wasn't just reflected in what I was eating. It was reflected in the fact that I wouldn't wear make-up, wouldn't make an effort with my hair and wouldn't do my laundry.

Can you believe that I wouldn't even light nice candles that people had gifted me because I was waiting to become one of those thin people who deserved to light a nice candle, sit in a nice environment, and be proud of themselves? Let's face it, you never see an advert featuring an overweight woman getting into a bath, moisturising, indulging in any kind of luxury, or enjoying a chocolate bar because it's delicious.

Something had started to shift and I started to entertain the idea of making the waiting room for weight loss a nicer place to hang out. Maybe, just maybe, it would be possible to dress up, swim, even eat in public, despite not being thin yet?

SHAHROO IZADI

Breaking the Pattern: When Self-Care Changed the Game

With this new insight, I decided to try an experiment: I would start acting as though I was never going to lose weight. So, I began lighting the candles I had been saving for the dinner parties that the thin version of me would throw. I started allowing myself to believe that my body, even though it wasn't thin yet, was worthy of taking a little more care of, even during periods of overeating. And I had no problem identifying what those choices would be, since I'd been making lists of them my whole life.

Admittedly engaging in self-care and making kinder choices for myself felt extremely unnatural, fake and silly at first. I realized how uncomfortable and unfamiliar it felt to treat my body nicely, when I still hated how it looked.

Once I started caring for myself as if I'd already lost weight (or as if I never would lose weight, which practically looked the same), I noticed that I felt much more deserving and capable of actually doing it. In fact, I found myself losing weight for the first time by accident. Moreover, I wasn't gaining it back. For the first time in my life I was achieving maintenance – because I wasn't eating as though food was being taken away from me and so there was no way to fail. Over time, my efforts to decouple self-care from food and body size started to make my periods of overindulgence shorter. Then, I found another missing piece of the puzzle – something that would help me not only lose weight but keep it off once and for all.

The Addiction Connection: Finding a New Framework

Around this time, I started working in the field of addiction as an assistant psychologist for the NHS. I was trained in how to support society's most change-resistant and highly addicted people: individuals with no support systems, who had multiple mental health diagnoses and who were attempting to change ingrained behaviors and dependency, against a backdrop of homelessness, unemployment, trauma and profound shame. This was when I started focusing on helping people who feel powerless over their own behaviors.

It was also the point at which everything shifted when it came to the way I approached weight loss. Just as terms and labels from therapy had previously helped me identify strategies that might help with issues like anxiety, entering the world of addiction helped me to truly see what it looks like when someone really wants to stop and just can't. Instead of looking up to celebrities who were constantly showing off their weight-loss results, I began to revere people who had simply stopped a self-destructive behavior. I remember my first patient telling me that he felt completely powerless over the heroin use that was ruining his life. He'd created a timeline to map the evolution of his dependency, one insidious, tolerance-building step at a time. He made it abundantly clear that, had he known the destruction his habit would bring, he would never have signed up for it – and that he would now do whatever it took to stop.

This man, and countless patients after him, who shared

honest details of their powerlessness with alcohol, gambling, sex, and so many other habits, reflected my relationship with food back to me far better than any nutritionist, dietitian or personal trainer. Every one of those patients described feeling so short-changed by substance abuse, and those who had maintained recovery for a while couldn't imagine anything but the clarity of abstinence following the chaos of their addiction. Listening to them made me realize that each of my own failed diets had left me with a stronger addiction to every aspect of the weight-loss cycle.

It wasn't long before I was able to perform the same tasks as a qualified recovery worker; this was partly because I loved every minute of my job and partly because I had started to see myself as an addict. I happily volunteered for late-night shifts and I took whatever I learned home and applied it to myself. I started to approach my inability to eat differently in the same way as an addict would approach using differently or not using at all. While exploring 12-step mutual aid groups, such as Alcoholics Anonymous, that were helping so many patients, I realized that I was not simply a 'food addict'. It turned out that during the decades of repeat dieting I had become addicted to both the 'high' of sugary foods and the 'benefits' of overeating something that is much more complicated to recover from.

Many overeaters don't just feel powerless when it comes to chasing the blissful hit of highly sugary food, they also come to learn that overeating to the point of discomfort in itself effectively numbs emotional pain and temporarily quietens shameful internal dialogue.

Creating My Own Version of Recovery

After leaving the NHS, I continued working on substance misuse in every capacity I could, and I've never looked back. I was trained in all the evidence-based motivational approaches used in hospitals, prisons, rehab facilities, and the community. As my work continued, it became clearer to me that these weren't just interventions for addicts.

Instead, the strategies being used were simple, reflective, behavioral change techniques focused on building the fundamental self-belief required to manage any habit more effectively (techniques I'll come back to in the last section of this book). So I used them to build on the gains I had made through my self-care routines and the feelings of self-worth they restored in me. By treating my struggle to maintain a healthy way of eating with the compassion, seriousness and respect I would give an addict who was struggling to stick to their programme, I lost eight stone in 18 months.

Eventually, I became a consultant and a trainer myself and travelled across the country, educating thousands of health and social care workers in how best to empower addicts to change for good. I started to develop habit-change workshops that incorporated (in a step-by-step process) everything I had seen to be helpful. Time after time, I delivered on my promise: *I will show you how to change any habit, without you even needing to share what habit you're here to change.*

SHAHROO IZADI

From Educator to Expert: My Mission Begins

Word started spreading that my workshops were effective and I was contacted by a highly respected journalist who was concerned about her binge drinking, but didn't want to stop drinking completely and wondered if I might be able to help. Historically, when it came to alcohol and other drugs, I'd only been tasked with helping someone stop altogether. But because I had already lost eight stone while still having to consume food – the substance I felt powerless around – I thought: *why can't I teach her to drink the way I've learned to eat?* Why not create guidelines that call abstinence two glasses of wine on a Friday night and that treat the third glass as a relapse?

Over a series of meetings, I spoke to her about how she could feel empowered by stopping when a behavior started taking more than it was giving. She published an article about our work together, which led to a literary agent reaching out and yet another pivot in my career – this time to author and coach.

My first two books, *The Kindness Method* and *The Last Diet*, were based on what I knew from my own experiences and from working in addiction therapy. And after my books were published, something extraordinary happened. I was inundated with messages from people who weren't necessarily looking for more answers, they just wanted to share their stories with me. They thanked me for the strategies I'd provided, but what truly resonated with them was my personal journey and how it enabled them to stop feeling they were stupid and weak.

HOW DIETS MAKE US FAT

Since then, I've devoted my life to understanding this problem. For well over a decade, during more than 10,000 hours of one-on-one conversations, I've been obsessively collecting stories, studying patterns, and refining approaches for the most resistant cases: the ones who have tried everything, have everything working against them, and can't stick to healthier eating patterns.

I've talked to thousands of people who were afraid to tell anyone else about what and how they eat when no one's watching. I've heard the tearful confessions of global leaders of industry who can manage complex careers but can't control themselves around a doughnut. I've analyzed the specific patterns that keep smart, disciplined people trapped in cycles of restriction and bingeing. This isn't just a career – it's a mission. And what I've now discovered goes way beyond conventional diet wisdom.

Chapter 2

A New Paradigm

Through collecting thousands of stories for well over a decade, I've discovered that there are two completely different types of dieters walking this earth. Two types with wildly different experiences, different needs, and different paths to healing. Yet we're all being sold the same recycled advice as if we're identical.

The first group is what I call the 'Too Much of a Good Thing' dieters. These are people for whom conventional advice actually works. When they put on a few pounds over the holidays, they simply dust off some sensible guidelines and get back on track. They view food as fuel and pleasure, not as a battleground of shame and desperation.

Then there's the second group: Sensible Sobriety Seekers – people doing what any sensible person would do in their situation. Like someone with alcoholism seeks sobriety from drinking, these individuals seek sobriety from eating, because eating nothing feels easier and safer than eating most foods, especially enjoyable ones. These people are caught in a psychological and biological hell that conventional diet wisdom not only fails to address but actively makes worse. This is what I call Restriction Addiction – developing a dependency on NOT eating because it's your best bet. You're not simply – or even at all – addicted to food. You're addicted to the control, silence and hope in its absence. Eating nothing has become genuinely easier than eating most things, because eating nothing is the only state where you're not bingeing, not obsessing, able to function. This pattern overlaps substantially with Atypical Anorexia Nervosa – meeting psychological criteria for anorexia while remaining at higher weight despite significant loss. The same psychological mechanisms applied, but different outcomes due to biological factors that kept forcing rebounds. This is why I call you Sensible Sobriety Seekers. You're seeking sobriety from food chaos through the only method that's ever worked: complete restriction. Like someone with alcoholism sensibly seeks sobriety from drinking, you're sensibly seeking relief from the loss of control that eating triggers. Given these two options, restriction or chaos, this becomes the most rational choice available.

I have observed, heard and read about this pattern time and time again in my practice; and what makes it so devastating is that there are so many obvious reasons why Sensible Sobriety Seekers are often invisible to researchers, healthcare practitioners, and even to the people experiencing it.

HOW DIETS MAKE US FAT

The Failure Legacy: When Each Diet Leaves You Heavier

In the early days of my professional work, I never managed to truly work out why I not only gained weight back after diets, but I gained more and more weight every year and after each attempt. It never quite made sense to me why every time I tried to get smaller, I only got bigger.

It wasn't until I questioned this compounding weight gain that I found an explanation that perfectly captured what I had experienced over many years, despite my repeated attempts to lose that weight – indeed, as it would transpire, *as a result* of my repeated attempts to lose weight.

I knew I was a 'yo-yo dieter', but compounding weight gain wasn't something I'd ever thought to consider. Yo-yo dieting involves fluctuations that can return to a baseline, but the additional challenge of compounding weight gain occurs when the regain phase consistently exceeds the initial weight loss, leading to a gradual increase. I was steadily gaining the extra weight for a reason and it became more significant each time. For me (and, I'd go on to learn, many other people), each failure left me more powerless around food and more in need of food as a coping strategy to deal with that failure.

In order to eventually lose weight, I had to unlearn a series of beliefs: beliefs about what it was worth putting myself through to be thin; beliefs about my unworthiness if I wasn't thin; beliefs about my ability to enjoy or appreciate my life if I was fat; beliefs that I couldn't be trusted to know how to eat because I wasn't even able to make the simple choices required to be thin. In other words, beliefs specifically embedded by diet culture.

Ultimately I lost eight stone by restoring my behavior to that of someone who ate as though it wasn't a moral choice; by training myself to behave like someone who wasn't on a diet. Or, as is now evident, someone who doesn't gain weight every year.

Since then, through continued exploration of my own history and thousands of conversations with clients, I've also come to recognize other, important dimensions of the problem that weren't on my radar when I began this work. They weren't even on my radar when I wrote my first two books. While my expertise in addiction psychology gave me the foundational tools to help people recover, it was my experience of hearing from readers and encountering the same patterns that made me realize that the problem was worse than I could ever have imagined and getting worse by the day.

The Systematic Pattern

I began to understand more about how Sensitive Sobriety Seeking follows a predictable pattern: the foundation is often laid in childhood through early messages that connect body size to worth, often before the person has developed any relationship with food as sustenance. This early programming can be particularly devastating because it happens before critical thinking develops. Children absorb these messages as fundamental truths about the world, rather than cultural beliefs that can be questioned. By the time they're old enough to think critically, the programming feels like unchangeable reality.

What starts as eating a bit less can escalate to increasingly extreme restriction attempts, each more desperate than the last. The body and brain can then adapt over time to protect against perceived recurring famine, becoming more efficient at storing fat and more sensitive to restriction with each cycle. A person's identity can become fused with the pursuit of thinness through restriction, making any approach that doesn't promise weight loss feel like giving up. They then fall through the cracks of research and treatment because they don't fit existing categories and are perpetually 'between attempts'.

Each cycle becomes more extreme: shorter restriction periods, more catastrophic rebounds, greater weight gain and deeper shame. What makes this progression so insidious is that every failure feels like evidence that the person needs to try harder, be more extreme, find a better diet. The system is designed to make failure feel like personal inadequacy, rather than systemic dysfunction, ensuring that people keep returning for more of what is really moving them further from what they want.

I also identified key factors that make some people more vulnerable to becoming a Sensitive Sobriety Seeker. In particular, differences that affect impulse control and reward processing, trauma histories that disrupt the body's stress response systems, and exposure to modern conditions (such as the availability of highly processed food, coupled with endless food advertising) all amplify these vulnerabilities. And the most crucial discovery? The invisible accelerant that determines who develops Sensible Sobriety Seeking and who doesn't comes down to one word: shame. This isn't just disappointment when the scale doesn't move. This is bone-deep, identity-level shame that transforms something as basic as eating into a moral emergency. It's a phenomenon I have observed in practically every person I've worked with, and I am going to return to it in depth in Part 2.

Many of the behaviors exhibited by this second group I've called Sensible Sobriety Seekers would traditionally be labelled as Binge Eating Disorder (BED), but what I've discovered in my clinical practice goes far beyond the standard criteria for BED. What I've been describing to you – this cycle of restriction and rebound that creates unprecedented conditions – engineered hyperpalatable foods, constant diet culture messaging, food environments overriding natural satiety signals: a perfect storm of conditions that has created an accelerated path to obesity that would have been impossible in any previous era. The combination of diet culture, engineered foods, chronic stress, and systematic shame has created a petri dish for Sensible Sobriety Seeking to flourish – and not only in those who are vulnerable to addiction.

The Game Has Changed

While the issues we are facing today are extraordinary and dangerously misunderstood, what I'll also show you is that the weight-loss game has been rigged from the start. You'll understand why you're not dealing with a 'willpower' problem: that, in fact, your struggles represent predictable responses to restriction. You'll understand that what's been happening to you could only happen in our time, with unparalleled intensity, and how the diet and food industry profits from keeping you trapped in this cycle. It's a business model that depends on failure because if diets worked permanently, the industry would collapse overnight. Instead, what's been created is the perfect product: one that provides temporary results, inevitable relapse, and a customer who blames themselves when it fails. It's ingenious and deeply harmful. Worse still, the very solutions you're being sold are really the cause of your problems.

Once you see how this system has been constructed around you, how your personal struggle is actually part of a much larger pattern affecting millions, everything changes. The shame lifts. The self-blame stops. And for the first time, real recovery becomes possible. So let's start by shining a light on a set of behaviors you may recognize – and explore why they are happening. Part 2 examines the bigger picture – the forces that created these patterns. Then Part 3 gives you the complete framework for breaking free and losing weight sustainably by addressing what's actually been driving the chaos.

PART 1

WHAT HAPPENS WHEN YOU DIET

Chapter 3

How You Know: Why Understanding Your Patterns is the Way Out

You've read the books. You've followed the plans. You've counted the calories, points, macros, or whatever is fashionable or repackaged as 'healthy' this decade. Yet here you are, possibly heavier than when you started, definitely more confused, and increasingly convinced that there must be something fundamentally wrong with you if you haven't managed to 'crack' this eating thing once and for all.

What I'm about to share is the first piece of a larger jigsaw that explains why you've found yourself trapped in this cycle despite your best efforts. More importantly, I will give you the information you need to create lasting change and lose weight for good. People who finally zoom out and clearly see their own patterns of behavior typically have the same revelation: *This explains everything I've been experiencing for years.* And with that understanding comes something even more valuable – a plan of action that doesn't rely on the approaches that have repeatedly failed. Understanding these mechanisms is essential for the sustainable weight-loss framework delivered in Part 3.

The Critical Behavioral Connection to Weight Loss

In this section of the book, I will detail five patterns that will help you start to understand why you're where you are today. What you're about to discover goes far beyond the conventional explanations you've probably been given before. We're not talking about motivation or 'willpower' issues. We're looking at something much more profound – a systematic disruption of your body's natural regulatory systems that has created patterns of behavior that would have been virtually unknown in any previous era of human history.

This method won't just make you feel better about your struggle, it will fundamentally change the way you approach weight management. Here's why: when you understand what's actually happening in your body and brain during the diet cycle, you will stop fighting against your biology and start working *with* it. This makes it much easier to manage your weight because you're no longer battling powerful biological forces designed to keep you alive. The dieters who succeed in the long term don't have extraordinary willpower: they're simply the ones who have learned to create conditions where less willpower is required. They've addressed the underlying mechanisms driving these patterns, rather than just fighting the symptoms.

But here's what most people don't realize: for many Sensible Sobriety Seekers, these mechanisms may have been so profoundly altered by repeated restriction that conventional approaches – even the 'sensible' ones – can no longer work. As I said in the previous chapter, what you're experiencing may be some-thing far more complex than standard eating challenges, something that requires a completely different understanding and an approach designed for your particular situation.

What You'll Discover

In each chapter I'll examine a different pattern in the chronic dieter's experience. First, I'll describe a specific struggle you're likely to be experiencing, whether it's the inability to stop once you start eating, constant thoughts around food, or the mysterious self-sabotage that occurs just when success seems within reach. Then I'll explore what you've probably been told is wrong with you: all the explanations diet culture has offered for your struggles, typically centered around character flaws, lack of willpower, or emotional issues.

These explanations aren't just wrong – they're actively harmful. What's happening operates at unprecedented scale and intensity – biological drives meeting an environment engineered to exploit them, combined with constant diet culture messaging impossible in any previous era. Think about it: your great-grandmother never had to navigate ultra-processed foods engineered to override satiety signals. She never encountered constant diet messaging or food advertising. She never lived in a culture that tied moral worth to body size.

As we progress, you'll begin to see how these behaviors interconnect and build upon each other. What emerges is a comprehensive picture of a condition that gets overlooked because it is largely invisible to both medical practitioners and the people suffering from it. You'll discover that your individual struggle is actually part of a much larger pattern. Then, in the final part of this book I will provide an approach to weight loss that is radically different from anything you've tried before, because it's designed for someone whose relationship with food has been fundamentally altered by dieting.

By understanding your patterns, you can address what's really driving your eating behavior and you can create conditions where losing weight and maintaining it finally becomes possible.

As your understanding deepens, something remarkable will happen. The shame that has been your constant companion will loosen its grip. You'll begin to see that you haven't been failing at diets – diets have been failing you. This isn't just a question of semantics; it's a profound shift in your mindset that will make you view food and your body through a new lens. You will realize that your struggles aren't random, personal or even unique. They're the predictable result of a system that has created the conditions for your Sensible Sobriety Seeking to develop at speed. Once you see it clearly – once you understand how your biology has been systematically disrupted and exploited – everything will change and you won't look back.

Chapter 4

The Myth of the Addictive Personality

*'Once I start, it's like I'm possessed.
I physically can't stop.'*

You take one bite of something you've been trying to avoid, maybe a biscuit, a slice of pizza, or a spoonful of ice cream. You've promised yourself you'll be 'good' today. (Let's be honest, you've barely eaten anything all day, surviving on black coffee and white-knuckling.)

That first bite tastes amazing. For a split second, you feel in control – you'll just have this one small portion and stop. But within seconds, something shifts. It can feel like a switch flipping in your brain. One bite becomes two, then three, then the entire packet. You're suddenly eating urgently, barely tasting the food anymore. It's like you're on autopilot – a part of you is watching yourself eat, unable to stop, while another part keeps reaching for more. Before you know it, you've eaten it all, and you're already planning to go out and buy more. You end up physically uncomfortable, disgusted with yourself, wondering what just happened to your self-control.

This pattern has been getting worse over time, hasn't it? And it feels intensely personal, as if it shows that there's something fundamentally broken about your character. You believe you must have an 'addictive personality'.

But what if I told you that this escalating pattern – this ever-shorter time between restriction and breakdown – is evidence of something more complex than simple food addiction? What you're experiencing isn't random personal weakness. It's the reshaping of your biology with each cycle, creating a far stronger current for you to swim against than the Group 1 'Too Much of a Good Thing' dieter.

What You Think Is Wrong

You've convinced yourself that your so-called 'addictive personality' makes you weak around food when others have no problem stopping at one biscuit. You secretly envy those people who can maintain perfect control over their eating. *At least they have discipline*, you think. You've tried to reach that level of control, but you always fail. What's more, you see evidence of your 'addictive personality' everywhere in your life. The way you tend to overdo things – not just with food, but perhaps with shopping, social media, work, or even exercise when you're on that health kick. The way you go all-in on new projects or habits, only to abandon them soon after. This all-or-nothing pattern seems to confirm what you've suspected about yourself all along.

Then there's the way you behave around food itself. Promising yourself 'just one bite' and then watching helplessly as you eat everything in sight. Hiding wrappers; eating in secret; feeling that powerful pull towards foods you're trying so hard to avoid. The behaviors feel exactly like what you've heard described as addiction: the cravings, the loss of control, the escalating consumption over time that never seems to satisfy. When you stumble across articles about dopamine – your brain's primary reward signal – and food addiction, everything seems to click into place. You think you recognize yourself perfectly when you read descriptions of sugar triggering the same parts of the brain that drugs do.

The withdrawal symptoms you experience when cutting out certain foods – headaches, irritability, overwhelming cravings – also all seem to confirm your self-diagnosis. This specific failure around food reinforces your deepest fear: that something in your brain chemistry is uniquely, fundamentally broken when it comes to eating.

The Hidden Reality

Here's the truth: there is no single personality trait that causes addiction. What appears to be an inherent character flaw is actually a complex interaction between your history, biology, and environment. What you're experiencing is your body's normal, predictable, hard-wired response to repeated cycles of restriction and bingeing. But this response is turbocharged by conditions that didn't exist for previous generations – the pressure to lose weight by restricting and the opportunity to gain weight by bingeing. Let that sink in for a moment.

The out-of-control eating you experience isn't happening despite your strict dieting efforts – it's happening *because* of them. Every time you severely restrict your food intake, you're unwittingly setting up the perfect conditions for bingeing. It's not a personal failing. It's a normal survival response. Anyone's body would react the same way under the same conditions.

What's Actually Happening

When you restrict food severely, even for short periods, your body can enter a state of perceived famine. It doesn't know this is voluntary. It doesn't understand concepts like 'diet' or 'bikini body'. It simply registers a dangerous shortage of incoming energy and responds accordingly, triggering a cascade of biological changes to protect you. Hunger hormones (like ghrelin) increase, while fullness hormones (like leptin) decrease. This creates a perfect storm inside your body – an environment where feeling satisfied with 'normal' portions becomes increasingly difficult. Your body is essentially running software designed for famine conditions while living in abundance. Think about those times you've been 'good' all day, then found yourself unable to stop eating once you start. It's your body correctly responding to signals screaming *EMERGENCY!* in your brain.

Restriction changes how your brain responds to food. The research is catching up to what's obvious clinically –

HOW DIETS MAKE US FAT

I've watched this pattern in hundreds of clients. Meanwhile, your brain's reward centers become more sensitive to food. What would give a normal eater a mild pleasure response now hits you with the force of an overwhelming compulsion. That first bite triggers a dopamine response – a chemical in the brain involved in reward and motivation. But here's the crucial difference: years of restriction-binge cycles have made your brain hypersensitive to this response. That's why that first bite feels so intensely good, and why it triggers such a powerful drive to keep eating.

Perhaps the most fascinating aspect of all this is what is happening to your executive function: the part of your brain involved in rational decision-making that has been temporarily overridden by the urgent need to survive. No amount of willpower can overcome this. It's like trying to think your way out of a sneeze.

All this happens while your metabolism is slowing dramatically. Your body becomes more efficient at storing energy after multiple restriction-binge cycles. This explains, from a basic evolutionary perspective, why each restriction-binge cycle leaves you heavier than before: your body is trying to protect you from what it perceives as recurring famines.

What's particularly striking is how these biological changes compound over time. For people who've been cycling through restriction and rebellion for years or decades, these adaptations can make it feel as if your biology works differently from that of someone who's never dieted. The longer this pattern continues, the more extreme and entrenched it becomes –

creating a compulsion that goes far beyond what most people understand as an everyday eating struggle.

As your body adapts to repeated restriction, your mind develops patterns that feel deeply personal but are actually predictable responses to the conditions you've created around food. After periods of severe restriction, your mind genuinely believes famine is imminent, creating an urgent 'eat now while you can' mindset as soon as food becomes available. This explains the frantic nature of binges – eating while standing up, barely chewing, sometimes not even tasting the food. It's not gluttony or lack of discipline. It's your brain responding with appropriate urgency the same way your ancestors would have after periods of involuntary famine.

Alongside this, you've developed a 'last supper mentality'. You have come to associate eating freely with pending restriction. It's that voice in your head during binges that says: *Might as well eat it all now since you'll be starting over tomorrow.* This explains the frantic quality of many binges – the sense that you need to eat everything right now, because tomorrow the opportunity will be gone.

This whole process creates a powerful pattern. The brief psychological relief of abandoning restriction after days of fighting hunger becomes a reward in itself. Your brain learns that eating brings the only available escape from the constant anxiety, hunger, and obsessive food thoughts that come with extreme restriction.

Perhaps the most insidious effect is the way your mind learns to categorize certain foods as 'forbidden', which gives them exaggerated importance and power. The more you try

HOW DIETS MAKE US FAT

to avoid these foods, the more your brain fixates on them, creating a pull that feels increasingly magnetic whenever they appear. For some people, this restriction-rebellion cycle becomes so deeply entrenched that it fundamentally rewires how they think about food, eating, and their own worth. Recognizing the psychological patterns described here is just the beginning of understanding what can happen when this cycle becomes a way of life rather than an occasional struggle.

Repeated dieting has also trained your brain to categorize eating behavior as either 'perfect' or 'failed'. These binary thinking patterns eliminate the mental space for moderation, making small indulgences feel like total disasters. You'll notice this in your internal dialogue when you eat something unplanned: *Well, I've already blown it for today!* The very idea of a minor deviation doesn't exist in your thinking – there's only adherence or collapse.

This all-or-nothing thinking becomes particularly entrenched when you have been cycling between restriction and rebellion for extended periods. What might start as simple diet rules gradually becomes a rigid psychological framework that makes moderate choices unthinkable.

Once you've broken a strict rule (having that first bite), you enter that 'what-the-hell' moment, where breaking a rule slightly feels equivalent to breaking it completely. This explains what's happening when eating one biscuit leads to eating the entire packet – not because you lack willpower, but because your brain has been conditioned to view any deviation as complete failure.

You may also experience restriction as rewarding, through

the sense of control and virtue it provides. This creates a psychological pendulum where the 'high' of perfect restriction swings inevitably to the 'low' release of complete abandon. But this sets up a psychological dynamic where the eventual breakdown feels like both failure and release – a pattern that can become intensely addictive in itself.

The Only Options Left

Given what's happening in your body and brain right now, you really only have a few options available to slow down your inevitable weight gain or weight regain, though none of them will solve the underlying problem. You could:

- Maintain periods of extreme restriction. This is probably what you're doing now: enduring short-term stints of highly restrictive eating. You know they'll inevitably end in loss of control, but at least they temporarily halt the weight gain. Without any stable middle ground, these restriction periods become your only tool for managing your weight, even though they're setting you up for the next binge. While no one would recommend this, what most people fail to understand is that this approach feels like the best strategy you have to prevent yourself gaining weight at speed.
- You might rely on a complete elimination of trigger foods. Since almost any manufactured product – typically foods high in sugars, salts, and fats and designed to be irresistible – triggers an uncontrollable

HOW DIETS MAKE US FAT

binge for you, avoiding entire categories of food completely might seem like your best chance at weight management. But this is almost impossible in today's food environment where we're constantly bombarded by advertising and these products are available literally everywhere. Yet this complete elimination feels like your only practical option when moderation seems impossible.

- Many people in your position turn to meal replacements to eliminate choice entirely. Given your current sense of overwhelm from food decisions, removing choice (by buying pre-packaged diet foods or shakes) may provide structure and make you feel safer. Or you might turn to appetite suppressants or weight-loss drugs that eliminate hunger, food choice and food noise altogether. Though you know this strategy is unsustainable in the long term, these products provide brief periods where your weight gain slows or reverses, giving temporary relief. Essentially you've resigned yourself to the idea that food will never represent joy for you again and that removing decisions about it is best for your mental and physical health.
- You could arrange your environment to limit exposure to trigger foods, acknowledging your current limitations while attempting to minimize their impact.
- You might schedule planned 'perfect' and 'off' days – formalizing a pattern you're already experiencing. This won't solve the problem but may reduce some of the shame around the inevitable cycles.

- You could also join Overeaters Anonymous or Food Addicts Anonymous. The structure and 12-step programme offered by these organizations treats your relationship with food as a true addiction requiring lifelong management, and this framework helps millions. But the required acceptance of 'powerlessness' reinforces your belief that you're fundamentally beyond repair from dieting, and the abstinence model can create more fear about a substance you still have to consume all day every day. When you inevitably eat a 'trigger food', your perfectionist brain interprets it as total failure, leading to massive shame spirals and bigger binges.
- You could transfer your 'addiction' to exercise, replacing food obsession with exercise compulsion, believing you're channelling your addictive personality into something healthy. But your all-or-nothing brain only knows one setting: extreme. You'll exercise for more than two hours daily, seven days a week, because that's what dieting taught you – if some is good, more is better. When injury or life prevents extreme exercise, you won't scale back to moderate exercise, you'll stop entirely, just like you do with food. Your brain only associates exercise with weight loss and punishment, so when you miss a few days, exercise feels pointless. The complete stop triggers both emotional eating (your old coping mechanism) and total exercise avoidance. When you're crying after a bad date at 11pm, you can't go straight to the gym,

so you're back to food as your only available comfort, often eating more because you feel guilty about 'failing' your exercise routine too.
- You could also chain smoke or vape. Nicotine suppresses appetite and gives you something to do with your hands when you feel 'possessed' by food thoughts. But you're just switching one compulsive behavior for another that damages your lungs. When you inevitably quit smoking, your appetite rebounds stronger than before and you're back to feeling 'addicted' to food, with added nicotine withdrawal symptoms making everything worse.
- You could try stimulant medication. These reduce the dopamine-seeking behavior that makes you feel 'possessed' by food thoughts; get you hyper so you're burning more calories from restlessness; and make you feel like you're full when you haven't eaten. But you're treating normal hunger and emotional needs as a medical condition requiring pharmaceutical management. When the medication stops working or you can't get it, the 'addiction' feels worse than ever because you've confirmed that you need drugs to control your eating habits.
- You could get gastric sleeve or gastric band surgery. If you're truly 'addicted' to food, surgically limiting your stomach capacity can make extreme bingeing physically impossible – even, as in my case, physically dangerous. But surgery doesn't change your compulsive relationship with food. You'll find ways

around the restriction through liquid calories, grazing, or stretching your pouch. When you regain weight despite surgery, you feel you've proved that your 'addiction' is so severe that even surgical intervention can't help you.

What You Actually Need

What you truly need is a complete reset of your relationship with food – one that addresses the biological and psychological patterns driving your loss of control while still supporting your desire to manage your weight.

First, you need to understand the crucial difference between true food addiction and what's happening to you. Your brain can respond to foods differently not because of an addictive personality, but because of the restriction-binge cycle you've developed. Understanding this difference frees you to target the actual mechanism instead of fighting a perceived character flaw.

You also need to see clearly why some people can stop at one biscuit. It's not that they possess greater willpower or discipline. It's that their brains haven't been sensitized by repeated restriction. Learning to distinguish between enjoying food and being controlled by it becomes essential. The difference isn't how much pleasure you get from food. It's the panic response your brain has developed to its availability after restriction. Seeing this distinction lets you dismantle the panic and eventually feel safe in enjoying the pleasure that food naturally provides.

HOW DIETS MAKE US FAT

Most importantly, you need to separate who you think you are from what's really happening inside your body. The behaviors you've previously attributed to a permanent 'addictive personality' are actually predictable biological and psychological responses to specific conditions you've created through repeated restriction. So separating identity from biology gives you the power to change those conditions and watch your behaviors transform.

But here's what you really need to understand: for some people, this pattern has become so deeply entrenched that standard approaches to 'food addiction' or even clinical eating disorder treatment aren't sufficient. When restriction and bingeing have been your primary relationship with food for years or decades, when your entire identity has become wrapped up in the pursuit of control through dieting, when shame about your body and eating has become fundamental to the way you see yourself, and you want to lose weight now more than ever, a completely different understanding and approach is required.

The restriction-binge cycle we've explored in this chapter is just the tip of the iceberg. What lies beneath is a complex interplay of modern food environments, cultural pressures, biological vulnerabilities, and psychological patterns that create something more challenging than most people – including many healthcare professionals – yet recognize.

You need to accept that when it comes to behavioral change, the path to success isn't to fight harder against these irresistible urges. It's changing the conditions that create those urges in the first place. But for those caught in the most extreme version of this pattern, this change requires you to understand forces and factors that go far beyond what we've discussed so far.

Chapter 5

The Information Prison

'I'm not sure what I'm allowed to eat anymore.'

You stand in the supermarket, paralyzed, in front of the yoghurt section. Low-fat or full-fat? Greek or regular? Sugar-free or fruit on the bottom? Your mind races through contradictory advice from every diet you've ever tried. The last plan said dairy was inflammatory and should be avoided entirely. The one before that recommended Greek yoghurt as a perfect protein-rich snack. The one before that insisted on fat-free varieties only. And wasn't there something about how artificial sweeteners might be worse than sugar?

Your trolley sits empty as other shoppers weave around you, seemingly unburdened by the mental gymnastics that have frozen you in place. This mental gridlock happens everywhere: at restaurants as you scan menus with mounting anxiety; in your kitchen as you second-guess every ingredient in every recipe; at social gatherings where a simple offer of food triggers an internal crisis.

What used to be simple – eating when hungry, stopping when full – has become a complex equation with too many variables and no clear solution. You've watched bananas move from a perfect healthy snack to a sugar bomb to be avoided, then to an acceptable but only-before-noon food depending on which diet you're following. You've reached the point where you rarely feel confident about any food decision. Instead, you cycle between rigid adherence to whatever plan you're currently following or complete abandonment when the rules become too confusing or too restrictive.

But here's what you may not have given due consideration to: this paralysis isn't just frustrating – it's actively feeding the restriction-rebellion cycle that's been trapping you for years. Foot chatter and confusion pushes you towards one of two extremes: either increasingly rigid rules (because uncertainty feels unbearable) or complete abandonment of all structure (because the rules have become impossible to follow). This pattern of swinging between desperate control and chaotic rebellion is creating something far more destructive than simple confusion about nutrition.

What You Think Is Wrong

You believe you've lost your fundamental ability to make sensible food choices. Where others seem to navigate eating with ease, you feel perpetually uncertain. You assume this reflects some personal deficiency in your judgment or intuition around food. *If I were smarter or more disciplined, I would just KNOW what to eat,* you think as you watch others casually make choices without the mental warfare you experience.

Maybe they're privy to some nutritional wisdom you've somehow missed? Maybe their bodies give them clearer signals? Whatever the reason, you're convinced that normal people don't experience this overwhelming uncertainty. It's not that you don't know what's healthy; it's that you don't know what's healthy for *you*, not least if you still want to lose weight. Despite having read countless diet books and articles, you still find yourself paralyzed by indecision in the simplest food situations. This disconnect between how much you've learned and how confused you still feel only reinforces your sense that something must be wrong with you. You're convinced that there must be one 'right' way to eat – one perfect system that would resolve your confusion if only you could find it and follow it correctly.

The gaps in your knowledge feel embarrassing. Even after investing thousands of pounds and countless hours in diet books, programmes, and expert advice, you still find yourself questioning whether brown rice is better than quinoa, if fruit contains too much sugar, or if that salad dressing will sabotage all your weight-loss efforts.

The Hidden Reality: Your Confusion is Manufactured

Here's the truth: you haven't lost your ability to make sensible food choices. You've been confused by design.

The contradictory information overload you're experiencing isn't accidental – it's the predictable result of a system that profits from your continued bewilderment and perpetual search for the next perfect diet plan.

Consider this stark reality: in the past five decades, dozens upon dozens of diet approaches have circulated, many directly contradicting each other. Low-fat, high-fat; low-carb, high-carb; eat for your blood type; eat for your DNA; don't eat after 6pm; only eat during an eight-hour window. These aren't subtle disagreements – they're often presented as direct opposites, each promoted with absolute conviction by experts with impressive credentials.

But this confusion isn't just frustrating you – it's destroying your ability not to abandon the whole thing and binge in chaos, let alone eat calmly and sensibly. Every contradictory piece of advice, every new food rule, every flip-flop between 'good' and 'bad' foods is pushing you deeper into the restriction-rebellion pattern that's been making you heavier with each cycle.

The endless parade of contradictory diet advice isn't evidence of evolving science – it often reflects marketing strategies more than science – and it keeps you in a constant state of uncertainty, always looking for the next solution. And each new solution requires you to restrict different foods, follow different rules, override your body's signals in different ways. Each attempt at finding the 'right' approach pushes you further from your natural ability to eat flexibly.

HOW DIETS MAKE US FAT

What's Actually Happening

This constant bombardment of contradictory advice has created a sophisticated psychological prison. Here's how it works . . .

- **The Paralysis Pipeline:** When faced with overwhelming food choices, it's common to seek certainty through increasingly rigid rules. The more confused you feel, the more appealing extreme restrictions become. Complete elimination feels safer than trying to navigate complex decisions. This is why you can cycle through dozens of moderate approaches but find yourself repeatedly drawn to the most restrictive plans – they promise an end to the exhausting uncertainty.
- **Dieter Dependency:** Being constantly told to override your body's wisdom in favour of external rules has disconnected you from your internal guidance system. You eat because it's 'time to eat', not because you're hungry. You finish your plate because that's the 'right portion,' not because you're satisfied. Many dieters become reliant on external rules and validation, finding it harder to trust themselves.
- **Binary Trap:** The all-or-nothing categorization of foods as 'good' or 'bad' has eliminated the nuanced middle ground where flexible eating exists. This creates an all-or-nothing approach where one unplanned biscuit triggers the thought: *I've blown it for today, might as well keep on eating and start*

fresh tomorrow. There's no room for the casual flexibility that allows typical eaters to have one treat and continue with their regular eating pattern.
- **The Perfect Storm Effect**: Each layer of confusion, each new restriction, each cycle of rules followed by rebellion has been building to something uniquely modern. What started as a simple desire to eat healthily has evolved into a complex psychological and biological pattern that would never have existed in previous generations, simply because they weren't dealing with the same confusion of diet information.

The Only Options Left

Given the information prison you're currently trapped in, you really only have a few options available:
- You could try to become a nutrition expert yourself, spending even more time researching and trying to resolve the contradictions. But this often leads to even more confusion as you discover that legitimate experts disagree fundamentally on basic questions and much of what's presented as established science is actually ongoing debate.
- You might choose one authority and follow them blindly, ignoring all contradictory information. This can provide temporary relief from decision paralysis but typically leads to increasingly extreme restrictions as you commit more deeply to approaches that eventually trigger biological rebellion.

HOW DIETS MAKE US FAT

- Live on meal replacement shakes and eliminate all the advice about what to eat by consuming complete nutrition in measured portions. But, by doing this, you're not learning how to navigate real food choices or conflicting information. When you go back to eating solid food, you have none of the skills needed to handle the overwhelming array of dietary advice and will likely regain the weight, plus more, while feeling more confused than ever.
- Or you could give up on any structured approach entirely, declaring that all nutrition advice is worthless. But this often leads to chaotic eating patterns that leave you feeling out of control and getting progressively heavier.
- You could get extensive food sensitivity testing. With so many diets claiming different foods are problematic, testing seems like a scientific way to find your personal 'bad' foods. But these tests often show false positives for foods that were never actually problems, giving you a new list of restrictions to follow rigidly. You end up with more dietary rules, not less confusion. Plus, as we know, if weight-loss drugs (where people lose weight whatever they eat, provided they're barely eating) have taught us anything, it's that eating less is ultimately the key.
- You could take food off the table altogether and turn to weight-loss injections to eliminate hunger. These medications suppress appetite so effectively that emotional eating urges should disappear entirely.

But they're pricey, and they don't teach you how to handle the underlying emotions. When you can't afford them anymore or they stop working, you're back to eating without any skills for handling feelings. In this situation, you will often end up even more trapped in the restriction-binge cycle because you feel you have 'failed' even with medical help.

None of these options addresses the real problem: that your natural relationship with food has been disrupted by forces much larger than your individual choices or knowledge gaps.

What You Actually Need

What you truly need isn't more or better information – it's freedom from the information prison itself. This means understanding how you got trapped, seeing clearly how the confusion serves interests other than your own, and beginning to rebuild trust in your body's wisdom while still supporting your health goals.

The path ahead isn't about finding the perfect nutrition plan or resolving all the contradictory advice. It's about understanding how modern conditions have disrupted the natural processes that once made eating simple and weight management automatic. Once you see this bigger picture clearly, everything changes.

Chapter 6

When Emotional Eating Stops Feeling Like Comfort

'I eat to change how I feel.'

You're three days into your new eating plan when your boss calls. That project you spent weeks on? They want major revisions by tomorrow. Your stomach tightens. Your shoulders creep towards your ears. Before you even realize what's happening, you're standing in the kitchen, hand buried wrist-deep in a box of cereal, mindlessly crunching as you stare blankly at the shelves.

This doesn't just happen when you're stressed. It's everything. Boredom on a Sunday afternoon? You find yourself opening the fridge. Argument with your partner? You reach for the ice cream before the conversation even ends. Loneliness at 10pm? That's when the takeaway delivery apps come out. Happy celebration? Food. Crushing disappointment? Food. Big feelings, small feelings, or the unsettling absence of feelings – food has become your universal response.

This pattern feels automatic, almost outside your conscious control. The pathway from feelings to food has become so well-travelled that it happens with frightening speed. Sometimes you're halfway through a bag of crisps before you even register what you're doing. It's as if your body has a direct line to food that completely bypasses any rational decision-making.

But what's truly maddening is that this emotional eating pattern seems to intensify with each diet attempt. The stricter your eating plan, the more powerfully your emotions trigger eating episodes. What started as occasional stress-eating evolves into an automatic response to virtually any feeling. You're not just gaining weight – you're losing your ability to experience emotions without immediately reaching for food. This isn't just emotional eating anymore; it feels more like addiction.

What You Think Is Wrong

You're convinced that you have a uniquely poor relationship with emotions. Other people seem to experience stress, sadness, or boredom without automatically reaching for food – so why can't you? It feels like a fundamental character flaw, some deep-seated emotional weakness that separates you from seemingly 'normal' people.

When you see a colleague calmly handle criticism without raiding the office biscuit tin, or watch a friend navigate a break-up without gaining a stone, it confirms your suspicion: there must be something emotionally deficient about you.

HOW DIETS MAKE US FAT

Normal people feel things without eating their way through them, or at least use proper drugs – like alcohol you think, as you order a takeaway after a difficult day.

You believe you lack basic emotional regulation skills that others were somehow born with or learned naturally. Maybe you missed some crucial developmental stage where people learn to self-soothe in healthy ways? Maybe you're just emotionally immature? Whatever the reason, you see yourself as unusually dependent on food to regulate your emotions.

Each time you eat in response to feelings, this belief deepens. You've tried everything: meditation apps, self-help books, even therapy, but nothing seems to break the automatic connection between feeling and eating. You suspect you might be using food as a substitute for something that's missing from your life – meaningful relationships, fulfilling work, or finding a deeper purpose.

The Hidden Reality: Restriction Breeds Emotional Eating

Here's the truth: your emotional eating isn't a character flaw or psychological failing. It's a predictable, and incredibly common, consequence of repeated food restriction. For most people who've been cycling through diets for years, this connection isn't coincidence – it's cause and effect. Here's what I've observed consistently across hundreds of clients: the restriction comes first, the emotional eating develops afterwards. The research on dietary restraint aligns with this – chronic restriction depletes emotional resources, disrupts mood regulation, heightens stress. Food becomes the obvious solution. The connection between dieting and emotional eating isn't just coincidental – it's come about specifically because, in your pursuit of weight loss, you have changed the way you feel emotionally by alternately restricting and overeating. Chronic restriction, followed by urgent, abundant consumption, can create a strong learned association between food and emotion. The longer someone has spent following various diets, the more pronounced their emotional eating often becomes. People with no dieting history typically don't develop the same types of intense emotional eating patterns, regardless of their psychological profiles or stress levels. Dieting history is a major factor, along with stress and individual differences.

Most eating is driven by factors other than physical hunger – emotions, environment, habit, stress. This becomes obvious when you pay attention to why people actually eat.

What's most remarkable is that this connection is universal. Emotional eating isn't limited to certain personality types or psychological profiles. It happens to virtually anyone who restricts food long enough. But here's what's truly disturbing: modern conditions have amplified this process. The combination of chronic restriction, engineered dopamine-boosting comfort foods that no one would ever label as healthy, and unprecedented stress levels has created emotional eating patterns that are far more intense and resistant to change. You are now no longer simply one of a handful of dieters; this is happening to more and more people. Comfort eating has become the rule, not the exception.

HOW DIETS MAKE US FAT

What's Actually Happening

When you chronically restrict food, several biological processes conspire to make emotional eating not just likely but inevitable . . .

- **Stress System Overload**: Restrictive eating can increase stress hormone levels, which make emotional triggers feel stronger. Any additional emotional trigger – even a minor one – can push your system into overwhelm. What might be a manageable emotion for someone else becomes physically intolerable because your stress response is already near its limit. You can observe this in the way small annoyances trigger disproportionate eating responses when you're dieting. The same minor frustration you might brush off easily when not restricting now sends you straight to the kitchen. This isn't emotional weakness – it's a body already at its stress threshold being pushed over the edge.
- **Brain Chemistry Depletion**: Restrictive eating can affect mood and reward systems, making the brain more responsive to the emotional effects of food. In effect, your body's natural mood stabilizers are running on empty. As these crucial neurotransmitters weaken, your emotional resilience deteriorates while your brain becomes hypersensitive to the mood-enhancing effects of food. Notice how strongly you crave carbohydrate-rich comfort foods – cakes, biscuits, crisps, pasta – during emotional moments,

and how quickly eating them provides emotional relief. This isn't coincidence; it's your brain efficiently addressing its chemical deficits.

- **Blood Sugar Chaos**: Restrictive eating can cause fluctuations in blood sugar, which can also impact emotional regulation. When blood sugar drops – common during dieting – the brain registers this as an emergency, triggering anxiety, irritability, and urgency. What feels like an emotional problem is often a physiological state driven by restriction-induced blood sugar fluctuations.

- **Ancient Survival Circuits**: Restriction can trigger powerful biological drives that don't distinguish between physical and emotional distress – they simply push you towards food whenever you're experiencing any feeling you would like to push away. From your body's perspective, stress is stress, regardless of whether it comes from dietary restriction, work pressure, or relationship problems. Your body has one solution to multiple problems: eat now, sort it out later.

- **The Control Paradox**: Many people use restriction itself as an emotional regulation tool – the control and structure provide temporary relief from anxiety and difficult emotions. When restriction inevitably breaks down, you're left without both your primary coping mechanism (restriction) and your back-up (food), creating 'perfect storm' conditions for emotional vulnerability. It's like using your life jacket as an anchor – the thing that's supposed to save you becomes the thing that drags you down when you need it most.

- **Forbidden Food Amplification**: Restriction transforms ordinary foods into potent emotional symbols. When foods are forbidden, their psychological significance grows precisely because they're restricted, making them increasingly compelling emotional management tools. Notice how the foods you turn to during emotional moments – the chocolate, ice cream, takeaways, biscuits – are typically the same ones you restrict most heavily. This isn't coincidence; it's evidence of how restriction amplifies their emotional power. Your body can come to associate certain foods with quick relief from emotional discomfort. Your brain isn't being irrational when it craves these foods during stress – it's seeking the most efficient solution to a biochemical problem created by restriction.
- **Pleasure Deficit**: Chronic restriction can reduce overall pleasure and satisfaction in life (as you well know). When food – one of the most fundamental sources of pleasure – becomes restricted, overall enjoyment can of course begin to diminish. This pleasure deficit makes emotional states harder to tolerate and increases reliance on the few remaining pleasure sources, often involving food binges. In other words: your drug of choice is becoming less effective as your need for it increases. This tolerance effect means you need progressively larger amounts

of food to achieve the same emotional relief, while simultaneously your capacity to enjoy other forms of pleasure decreases. Activities that used to bring joy – socializing, hobbies, accomplishments – feel flat and unsatisfying compared to the intense but temporary relief provided by food.

The Only Options Left

Given this restriction-driven emotional eating pattern, your current options are severely limited:

- You could try to develop better emotional coping skills while maintaining your restriction patterns. But this typically fails because the restriction itself is generating much of the emotional volatility and creating the biological drive towards emotional eating.
- You might attempt to eliminate all emotional triggers from your life, creating a highly controlled environment where you're less likely to be triggered into eating. But this leads to an increasingly constrained existence that becomes its own source of stress and emotional difficulty.
- Or you could accept emotional eating as inevitable and try to minimize damage through portion control or choosing 'healthier' comfort foods. But this rarely works because the biological and psychological drives we've described override conscious portion decisions. Trying to control portions during emotional eating episodes is like trying to negotiate with a tsunami.

HOW DIETS MAKE US FAT

- You could use ice baths or cold showers to 'reset' emotions: these techniques provide temporary relief from emotional intensity and might reduce stress eating in the moment. But they become another external dependency rather than building internal emotional regulation skills. When you're upset at work and can't take a cold shower, you're back to food with even more shame because your 'advanced' coping strategy 'failed'.
- You could go to bed early every time you feel emotional: sleep avoids night-time emotional eating and removes you from trigger situations. But you're teaching yourself that you can't handle emotions without escaping them. When you're stressed during the day and can't go to bed at 2pm, you're left with no coping skills so you default to food. You never learn that you can actually sit with difficult feelings and let them pass naturally.
- You could replace food with shopping when you are feeling emotional: the satisfaction you get from purchasing might satisfy the same need that food was meeting. But you're still avoiding learning how to self-regulate emotions – you're just switching from: 'I need food to feel better,' to 'I need to buy some-thing to feel better.' When your credit cards are maxed out and you're feeling anxious about money at midnight, you can't exactly go shopping, so you're back to food as your only available comfort.
- You could transfer emotional regulation to alcohol or

marijuana: these substances numb emotions effectively and might reduce emotional eating initially, but these substances also impair your judgment and lower inhibitions around food. When you're high or drunk, years of diet-trained restriction often leads to massive 'what-the-hell' eating episodes. Plus when you're sober and anxious from substance use, your brain defaults to food as the most familiar emotional regulator.

- You could try taking sleeping pills to avoid evening emotions and eating: medication helps you sleep through potential emotional eating times and avoid difficult feelings. But you're literally medicating yourself unconscious. When you can't take pills, or when emotions hit during the day, you're completely helpless. The pills reinforce your belief that emotions are too dangerous to experience while you're awake.
- Or you could take antidepressants or anti-anxiety medications to stop emotional eating: if medications stabilize your mood, you should naturally stop turning to food for emotional regulation. But many psychiatric medications have increased appetite as a side effect. More importantly, when life stress hits or the medication stops working, your years of not practising emotional regulation mean your brain immediately defaults to food. The medication becomes a crutch that prevents you from developing actual coping skills.

None of these approaches addresses the fundamental problem: that weight gain, body image and powerlessness is creating and amplifying the emotional eating pattern. If you reduce your emotional need for food as a coping strategy, or you find other coping strategies, you're still going to exist as a fat person in a body you dislike, feeling out of control. And so long as that underlying body hatred and food powerlessness remain, you'll still be vulnerable to using food for emotional regulation. In other words, you are still going to feel stressed out about being fat.

What You Really Need

What you truly need is a comprehensive approach to breaking the restriction-emotional eating cycle while supporting your weight management goals. You need to understand the biological connection between restriction and emotional eating. Recognizing that this pattern stems from predictable physical mechanisms rather than emotional weakness provides the foundation for effective change. This isn't about excusing emotional eating; it's about accurately identifying its causes so you can address them successfully.

You also need to stabilize those physical systems that influence emotional regulation. Establishing consistent eating patterns that can prevent blood-sugar crashes, hormonal fluctuations, and nutrient deficiencies creates the biological foundation for improved emotional-management without such heavy reliance on food. Alongside this, you'll need to build a diverse emotional management toolkit. Developing and practising non-food coping strategies that provide similar relief to emotional eating gives you viable alternatives.

However, these strategies will only be effective if they are implemented alongside changes to the restriction patterns that drive emotional eating in the first place – to acknowledge that food is a solution, not a problem.

You need gradual exposure to emotional experiences without food management. Through the practice of handling progressively more challenging emotions without immediately reaching for food, you can rebuild confidence in your natural capacity to regulate your emotions. Understanding this mechanism is essential for sustainable weight loss because until you address why you're using food emotionally, no eating plan will stick. Part 3 gives you alternative coping tools so food stops being your primary emotional regulator, which is when lasting weight loss becomes possible.

Chapter 7

When Your Food Landscape Shrinks

'I can only lose weight if I isolate myself.'

Your kitchen has become a carefully managed territory, with clear no-go zones. You daren't keep certain foods in the house – biscuits, crisps, ice cream, chocolate, bread – because their mere presence feels like a ticking time bomb. It's not a question of *if* you'll break down and eat them all at once, it's *when*.

What seems simple for others – having a packet of biscuits in the cupboard for weeks and eating one occasionally – feels impossible for you. If those biscuits cross your threshold, they won't survive the night. You know this with absolute certainty because it's happened countless times before.

This problem extends beyond your home. You have routes through the supermarket that deliberately avoid the bakery and snack aisles. You take the long way around the office to bypass the break room when doughnuts are delivered.

You've developed elaborate strategies for social events: eating beforehand so you won't be hungry around the buffet table, positioning yourself far from the food, keeping your hands occupied with a drink.

The most frustrating part? These aren't even foods you particularly love. Some of your trigger foods are items you'd rate as merely okay if judging on taste alone. Yet they hold this mysterious power over you. Once they're available, they become irresistible, regardless of hunger, fullness, or even enjoyment.

But here's what's becoming increasingly clear: this pattern is getting worse over time. Foods that you could once keep in the house occasionally are now completely off-limits. The list of forbidden foods keeps expanding. What started as avoiding obvious 'junk foods' has extended to items like bread, fruit, even nuts. Your world is shrinking as more foods become too dangerous to have around.

This isn't just about individual foods anymore – it's about a fundamental transformation in how your brain responds to the mere presence of anything you've tried to restrict or anything that is not objectively helpful for weight loss. You're not just avoiding specific items; you're living in a state of constant vigilance against your own appetite. And with each restriction cycle, this vigilance needs to become more extreme just to maintain the same level of control. It's exhausting and all-consuming, leaving fewer cognitive resources available for everything else in your life – work, relationships, creativity, joy.

HOW DIETS MAKE US FAT

What You Think Is Wrong

You believe you're inherently weak around certain foods when others have no problem keeping them around. You watch roommates, partners, or family members casually ignore the ice cream in the freezer for days while you can think of nothing else until it's gone. This selective vulnerability feels like profound evidence of your broken willpower.

There are moments when someone offers to leave tempting leftovers at your house, and you have to awkwardly refuse, knowing full well what would happen if they did. There are times when you can't go to a restaurant because, while other people can just order food based on what they fancy, you don't remember the last time you ate out and it didn't trigger a downward spiral. The same goes for birthdays, weddings, gatherings with friends that you are prepared to forego in order to maintain the momentum you've achieved on your diet. Your thinking? *I wouldn't enjoy myself anyway unless I'm thin, so why risk it?* Or worse, there are times you've assured someone (and yourself) that you can handle having that chocolate in the cupboard, only to devour it all minutes after they leave, unless you cover it in washing-up liquid to stop yourself putting it in your mouth.

Each incident reinforces the shameful conviction: you simply cannot be trusted around certain foods. More than that, you cannot be seen to eat because anyone observing you would see that the way you eat is unhealthy and your now tiny world is unhealthy too. It would be heartbreaking for a loved one to see how fearful and powerless you feel around food and how restrictive you are being. Little do they know that your world becomes even smaller every time your plan backfires, and you lose further trust in yourself.

You believe your only option is isolation. Since the risk has repeatedly proven to be not worth taking, you've resigned yourself to the idea that life is on hold until you are thin and the solution is complete control over your environment. This represents a profound loss of agency over your own life. You've essentially put yourself under house arrest, with parole conditional on achieving a body size that your restriction-damaged metabolism makes increasingly difficult to reach.

The Hidden Reality: Losing Won't Give You the Control You Crave

Here's the truth: your inability to feel calm when exposed to risky food situations or to trust yourself in different contexts, let alone in unforeseen and unpredictable contexts, is a direct result of diet culture creating a self-fulfilling prophecy. Through years of dieting and a growing list of 'bad' foods, you have to come to associate not only foods but a variety of physical settings with an inability to trust yourself.

Since so many of these will now have become associated with a final binge (because even the healthiest of gatherings will not limit the menu to celery), you can't be blamed for believing: *I've not been able to do this/go there/see this person without weight gain and self-loathing.*

HOW DIETS MAKE US FAT

What's Actually Happening

With each diet your world is becoming smaller and the trust that you have in yourself is being eroded. The more you isolate, the lonelier and more ashamed you feel and the more extreme your behaviors become. Because you can't explain the powerlessness you feel around food, it becomes easier not only to eat nothing, but to go nowhere until you are thin. Furthermore, you place no importance on your quality of life outside of your body size and where you are in your weight-loss journey.

Because of the anxiety you feel in these contexts, you are constantly making associations that reinforce the feeling that socializing is not fun until you're thin. Instead, every occasion – be it a party, restaurant or cake at work – feels like a source of panic and shame. This won't stop you from losing weight, but it will cause you to engage in a form of self-harm that no one would want to see you go through.

Each time you isolate yourself, your mind is being rewired to link certain situations to danger, as well as building new limiting beliefs about yourself. Not enjoying yourself then becomes a self-fulfilling prophecy – not just because of your body size but, as you see it, your greed, laziness, and evident self-hatred. The longer this goes on and the bigger you become, the less visible you want to be, both physically and in the way you behave around food. This is building towards something that goes far beyond everyday challenges with certain foods. It represents a breakdown of your natural ability to coexist peacefully with food in your environment and enjoy your life.

The Only Options Left

Your options seem severely limited:
- You could stop eating at restaurants or attending social events entirely: avoiding situations where you can't control every ingredient and portion seems like the safest approach. But you then develop a sense of powerlessness that extends far beyond food. You know you're always one dinner invitation away from losing control, so you start declining invitations. This powerlessness creeps into other decisions: *I might be able to handle that challenging project, but I can't even sit through a restaurant meal without panicking about the bread basket.*
- You could decide only to socialize with other people on restrictive diets: surrounding yourself with others who follow similar food rules provides support and eliminates peer pressure to eat 'normally'. But that means you're creating an echo chamber that reinforces your disordered thinking about food. When one person falls off the wagon, it often triggers everyone else to abandon their restrictions too. You never learn to navigate everyday social eating situations.
- You could isolate yourself to somewhere remote with limited food access: if ultra-processed foods aren't available, you can't be tempted by them. But isolation creates profound loneliness and boredom which are major emotional eating triggers. When you eventually return to civilization or get food delivered, your brain

drives you to eat everything you've missed. The period of forced restriction often leads to more intense food obsession and bigger binges than before.

- You could order pre-prepared meals to control all food decisions: having pre-prepared food removes all food choices and temptations from your daily life. But it's expensive and doesn't teach you any skills for real-world eating. When you can't afford the service anymore, you're completely helpless around food decisions and likely to regain weight rapidly while dealing with the financial stress.
- You could tell people you have serious medical food restrictions: lying about allergies or medical conditions gives you an excuse to avoid eating in uncontrolled situations. But maintaining the deception creates anxiety and damages relationships when people discover the truth. Plus you reinforce the idea that 'normal' foods are dangerous to you, making every social eating situation feel like a medical emergency.
- You could move back in with loved ones who monitor your eating. That might help you avoid immediate problems, but it infantilizes you and creates power struggles around food. You never learn adult coping skills, and the resentment often leads to secret eating and rebellion when you're out of their sight. The dependence on external control also makes independent eating feel impossible.
- You could visit residential weight-loss facilities repeatedly (or what we casually referred to in the

1990s as 'fat camps'): these programmes have full control over meals while you're there. But you're not learning how to navigate real-world food situations, social pressure, or stress. When you return home, the weight comes back because your environment and skills haven't changed. Each return trip reinforces the idea that you can't handle everyday life on your own.

None of these options fundamentally changes your relationship with your environment or your ability to maintain any weight loss. In fact, the more no-go zones you collect, the more these risky environments will look like your risky list of foods, and it will echo the same pattern. The second you are not able to control anything, your anxiety levels will become intolerable and you'll rebel. You'll think: *I'm an adult and I can do what I like.* Essentially, you become a rebel without any cause.

What You Really Need

You need to intentionally collect evidence of your ability to make new choices in currently risky environments. These choices need to reflect the choices you would have made had diet culture not hijacked your mind and your body.

You need to accept this truth: thinness alone won't automatically restore healthy behaviors. Neither will 'common sense'. Ingrained patterns require systematic unlearning through repeated practice.

HOW DIETS MAKE US FAT

Just like mastering anything, practise through repeated exposure – along with gathering compelling proof of your ability to make something easier and a context less scary – will enable you to keep up any plan.

You need to treat this as skill-building and restoration. Just because we're talking about food, there is a tendency to trivialize and under-estimate the task of changing how you eat. You may think it should be simple but simple doesn't mean easy. Much like someone who was taught to drive incorrectly from the first day they got behind the wheel, your default habits need to be unlearned until autopilot looks very different.

Chapter 8
The Self-Sabotage Trap

*'Every time I make progress,
I find a way to ruin it.'*

You've been here before, haven't you? Three weeks into your new eating plan, the scales are finally moving in the right direction. Your clothes feel a bit looser. You're starting to believe that maybe – just maybe – this time will be different. Then it happens. Without warning, without intention, you find yourself in a drive-through, ordering enough food for three people. Or you're standing in your kitchen at midnight, eating leftovers straight from the container; or buying and consuming an entire pack of biscuits you swore you'd never bring into the house again.

The specifics change, but the pattern is brutally consistent: just when success seems within your reach, you do something that completely derails your progress. The weight piles back on – often with a few extra pounds as a parting gift – and you're left wondering what's wrong with you.

This isn't just the occasional slip-up. It's a predictable cycle that has repeated throughout your life. You make progress, get close to your goal, and then, almost as if something inside you can't tolerate success, you undo everything you've worked for.

And here's what's most disturbing: this pattern seems to intensify over time. What used to take months of progress before self-sabotage struck now happens after just weeks. Your body's resistance to weight loss appears to be getting stronger, more sophisticated, more automatic with each attempt. You're not just struggling with self-sabotage – you're experiencing an escalating biological rebellion that becomes more powerful with each diet cycle.

What You Think Is Wrong

You believe you must have some deep-seated psychological issue that makes you sabotage your own success. Maybe you're subconsciously afraid of how your life might change if you reached your goal weight? Maybe you don't believe you deserve to be thin? Maybe you've become so accustomed to your identity as someone who struggles with weight that success feels threatening to your sense of self?

These suspicions haunt you, especially in quiet moments after another round of self-sabotage: *Why would I do this to myself?* you wonder late at night. *Do I secretly want to be fat? Am I afraid of success? Do I somehow need to struggle to feel normal?* You search your psyche for the hidden emotional blockage that must be preventing your success.

You suspect there might be secondary gains from remaining overweight that you're not consciously aware of – perhaps being heavier provides protection from unwanted attention, from expectations, or disappointment.

You wonder if you have some form of self-destructive personality trait that extends beyond food. You notice that when things are going well in other areas – relationships, career, finances – you sometimes make choices that undermine your progress there too. This pattern of snatching defeat from the jaws of victory feels like a fundamental character flaw, something written into your DNA.

You believe that successful people must have something you lack: stronger willpower, better self-discipline, or a healthier psychology. The fact that you can't maintain progress despite genuinely wanting to lose weight seems like definitive proof that you're simply not cut out for success in this area. You're convinced that if you could just understand the psychological root of your self-sabotage, if you could identify and resolve whatever emotional issue is driving this behavior, you could finally break the cycle and achieve lasting weight loss.

The Hidden Reality: You're Fighting Your Body's Weight Defence System

Here's the truth: you may well be sabotaging yourself in certain areas of your life due to deeper reasons like low self-esteem, and that is worth exploring. That said, if weight loss appears to be the only area where you are self-sabotaging, this means you have come to connect eating with the visible impact it will have on your body. This has been happening to such a degree and for so long that you genuinely believe that wanting to see those scales drop is important enough to override hunger.

This isn't about sabotage or, even if it is now, it didn't start that way. If your repeated failure and a body you hate has, over time, made you feel unworthy of the gift of thinness then it is possible that your self-sabotage has become more entrenched, but it wouldn't have got there without diet culture.

Your body defends a particular weight range – your set point. Your body naturally tends to resist long-term weight loss, working to restore your body to a range that its used to maintaining. When you lose weight below this range, your body initiates a coordinated response to bring your weight back up, regardless of your best intentions.

This defence system operates on multiple levels simultaneously: hormonal, neurological, metabolic, and psychological. It's not some vague emotional issue – it's a concrete biological reality with measurable effects that can override even the strongest resolve. You are facing the most challenging possible conditions for behavioral change – making a decision today in good faith that it will deliver tomorrow, when there is no guarantee of any long-term gain. This is delayed gratification applied to a completely different domain in your life, and one that has been totally informed by diet culture to further the level of disruption.

What's Actually Happening

When you lose weight, your body launches a coordinated biological rebellion aimed at restoring lost weight . . .

- **Hormonal Warfare:** Hormones that signal fullness – like leptin, GLP-1, and peptide YY – decrease. Studies tracking dieters over multiple years show these hormonal adaptations persist long after weight loss, creating sustained biological pressure towards weight regain. This might be why overwhelming hunger and food preoccupation seem to emerge just as you're making good progress. It's not emotional weakness – it's a hormonal response specifically designed to restore lost weight. The further below your set point you go, the more aggressively your body fights to conserve energy and the sooner sabotage seems to occur. The longer this goes on, the more it reinforces your core belief that you are someone who throws in the towel as soon as you've gained a bit of momentum.
- **Mental Exhaustion:** Then there's the mental breakdown. While the fundamental drivers of self-sabotage are biological, they manifest through specific psychological experiences that feel intensely personal but are actually predictable responses to weight loss. Long periods of food restriction wear down mental energy, making impulse control feel much harder. The mental energy required for constant food decisions eventually becomes unbearable. This isn't character

weakness – it's cognitive depletion, a well-documented phenomenon that affects everyone under conditions of prolonged self-control.

- **Reward Erosion**: Over time, the thrill of seeing the scales move diminishes while restriction continues to feel more uncomfortable, making setbacks more likely. More and more false starts at higher and higher weights start to create earlier and more frequent sabotage, as even success has come to be associated with failure.
- **Progressive Intensification**: Each repeated diet makes it harder to maintain progress, as your body and habits increasingly resist long-term change. You used to achieve months of progress before triggering self-sabotage but it now happens after weeks. Your biological rebellion is learning, adapting, and becoming more efficient at protecting you against weight loss.

The Only Options Left

- You could eat all your meals in front of a mirror: watching yourself eat forces constant self-awareness and might shame you into eating less. But for someone already triggered by body shame, this becomes psychological torture. Your brain alternates between thoughts of *I look disgusting eating this* (leading to restriction) and *I hate looking at myself* (leading to emotional eating for comfort). The mirror

HOW DIETS MAKE US FAT

eating often becomes so distressing that you start avoiding meals entirely or eating in secret.

- You could put 'fat photos' of yourself everywhere as motivation: visual reminders of your larger body might shame you into maintaining weight loss. But constant exposure to images you hate increases depression and self-loathing. Shame powerfully predicts both emotional eating and binge eating, creating a direct pathway to weight cycling, because it drives stress eating and leads you to give up entirely when you inevitably have imperfect eating days.

- You could weigh yourself multiple times per day: obsessive monitoring might keep you hyper-aware of every fluctuation and motivated to course-correct immediately. But normal fluctuations (from water, hormones, and digestion) create daily emotional rollercoasters. When the scales don't move or go up despite 'perfect' eating, you often give up entirely or restrict even more dangerously. The obsession with numbers leaves you unable to judge progress by how you feel or function.

- You could use 'portion shaming' plates and utensils: eating off plates labelled 'Mum Jeans Vs Skinny Jeans' or using vibrating forks that punish fast eating might shame you into better habits. But these tools turn every meal into a moral judgment on your appetite and eating speed. Your perfectionist brain becomes obsessed with eating only skinny-jeans portions and avoiding fork vibrations, making meals stressful performances rather than nourishing experiences.

- You could set up punishment systems for 'bad' eating: consequences like extra exercise, donating money, or public shaming when you eat forbidden foods might deter overeating. But punishment increases cortisol and makes food more appealing through rebellion psychology. The stress of constant self-monitoring often triggers more emotional eating, and the punishment reinforces the idea that you're fundamentally bad around food.
- You could ask friends to shame and monitor your eating: external accountability through friends policing your food choices might provide motivation through social pressure. But it damages relationships and makes you afraid to eat around others. Friends eventually get tired of being the food police, leaving you feeling more isolated and likely to eat emotionally. The social shame often triggers more secretive eating behaviors.
- You could practise constant body-checking during meals: pinching your stomach, checking your reflection, or monitoring how clothes fit while eating might keep you motivated to eat less. But this hyper-vigilance turns every eating experience into a body-shame session. Your brain can't focus on hunger, fullness, or satisfaction because it's busy cataloging all the ways your body is 'wrong'. This often leads to either mindless overeating to escape the body

awareness or severe restriction to punish the body you're monitoring.
- You could follow extreme 'fitspiration' accounts for daily shame motivation: constant exposure to idealized bodies and harsh motivation might shame you into maintaining your weight loss. But the comparison trap becomes addictive and destructive. When you can't maintain impossible standards, you feel like a complete failure. The constant comparison often leads to more extreme restriction attempts followed by bigger binges, plus depression and body dysmorphia that make weight management even harder.

What You Really Need

You need to stop expecting an aspirational dress size to enable you to tolerate hunger. Instead you need to create space for the reality that even if you had never been on a diet, changing habits – not least when it comes to food – is difficult and would be difficult for any human being.

You need to realize that it is your association that has turned the discomfort of imperfection in the pursuit of eating differently into sabotage. Eating and body size are so closely enmeshed that you haven't factored in how difficult embedding any new habit is. Essentially you need to get better at eating differently, not get better at getting thin. That way you will factor in that being on a learning curve that reminds you it is impossible to be perfect from day one.

Chapter 9

The Knowledge-Action Gap

*'I know exactly what to do –
I just can't make myself do it.'*

You're not lacking information. You could write a doctoral thesis on nutrition at this point. You know which foods are 'good' and which are 'bad'. You understand calories, macros, portion sizes, and meal timing. You've read the books, followed the experts, and accumulated more knowledge than most healthcare professionals. And yet, despite all this knowledge, you still can't consistently do what you know you should.

You make detailed meal plans on Sunday, but abandon them by Tuesday. You set clear intentions in the morning, then find yourself eating things you never planned by the evening. You identify all your triggers and patterns, then watch yourself fall into them anyway, as if you're observing someone else entirely.

It's this disconnect between knowing and doing that makes you question your fundamental character. If you genuinely want to lose weight, and you absolutely know how to do it, why can't you just follow through? This pattern extends beyond occasional slips. It's a persistent, distressing gap between your intellectual understanding and your actual behavior. You find yourself repeatedly making choices that directly contradict what you know would support your weight-loss goals, then beating yourself up afterwards for your apparent inability to act on your own knowledge.

But one thing is becoming increasingly obvious: this gap between knowing and doing is getting wider over time. Knowledge that once translated into action – at least temporarily – now seems completely disconnected from your behavior. It's as if your brain has two separate operating systems that can no longer communicate with each other.

What You Think Is Wrong

You believe you must have some profound weakness of character – a fundamental lack of discipline or follow-through that separates you from successful people. When you see others putting the same common sense into practice, you assume they must have some inner strength that you simply don't.

Each time you abandon your carefully crafted plan, this belief deepens. It's further 'evidence' that you simply don't have what it takes. When you read those endless success stories online, you focus on the person's determination and discipline. *I just don't have that mental toughness,* you think.

Your continued inability to follow their example feels

like evidence that you are stupid, haven't tried hard enough, haven't found the right approach, or simply don't want it badly enough.

The Hidden Reality: When Your Brain Splits in Two

The gap between your knowledge and your actions isn't a character flaw or a psychological issue. It's the predictable result of trying to use conscious decision-making in conditions it was never designed to handle.

Your brain's decision-making evolved in a food environment radically different from today's. The disconnect you experience between knowing and doing isn't evidence of weakness – it's evidence of normal brain function encountering an abnormal environment that's been specifically designed to override rational thought and natural primal responses.

People who appear to successfully bridge this gap aren't superior in willpower or discipline, they've probably just structured their lives to minimize the conditions that create the gap in the first place. They're not better at pushing through – they're better at creating environments where less pushing is required. But here's what's truly disturbing: modern conditions have made this gap wider and more difficult to bridge than ever before. You're not just dealing with the standard challenges of following through on plans – modern food environments make unhealthy choices the easiest option, requiring no effort, no planning, no decision-making.

What's Actually Happening

Your brain operates through two systems: System 1 is fast, automatic, emotional. It makes split-second decisions without conscious thought. System 2 is slow, deliberate, rational. It requires conscious effort and mental energy.

- **Planning**: Your reflective, rational system that processes nutrition information, sets goals, and makes meal plans. It operates slowly, requires mental energy, and thinks in terms of long-term consequences. This is the part of your brain that knows chocolate cake isn't the best choice for your weight-loss goals.
- **Acting**: Your automatic, intuitive system that executes moment-to-moment food decisions. It operates lightning-fast, prioritizes immediate rewards, and responds to environmental cues without conscious thought. This is the part that makes it harder for you to stop treating a craving as a command. You experience this split when you find yourself reaching for foods you explicitly decided to avoid.
- **Mental Energy Depletion**: Thoughtful decision-making requires significant mental energy to override automatic responses. As this limited resource gets depleted throughout the day, due to work stress, decision fatigue, and emotional demands, your brain naturally shifts towards automatic processing that prioritizes immediate rewards over long-term goals. You notice this pattern when your food choices deteriorate as the day progresses: your morning plans falling victim

to mental energy depletion in the evening. This isn't random failure – it's predictable mental resource depletion that affects everyone, not least those who have been stressing about what to eat and not to eat.

- **Stress Override**: When you're stressed, your brain automatically narrows attention towards immediate concerns and away from long-term goals. This neurological shift happens automatically, regardless of your conscious desires, which explains why stressful periods consistently undermine your eating plans despite your knowledge remaining perfectly intact.
- **Environmental Hijacking**: You form strong associations between environmental cues and eating behaviors through repeated experience. These associations trigger automatic responses that bypass conscious thought entirely, activating behavior before you can even think about it. While the fundamental problem is neurological, it's activated by specific environmental conditions that have been engineered to maximize the gap between knowing and doing and create fewer steps between an unhelpful thought and an unhelpful action.
- **Decision Overload**: Modern environments require you to make dozens of food decisions daily and expose you to an unprecedented range of options. Each decision depletes your limited mental resources until automatic processing inevitably takes over, regardless of what you know about nutrition. You experience this as the exhausting feeling of constantly

having to make 'good' food choices throughout the day. This exhaustion isn't laziness – it can be the cognitive burden of navigating far more decisions than your brain was designed to process.

- **Engineered Temptation**: Many modern foods are specifically designed to override your planning brain and trigger automatic consumption. Ultra-processed foods – things like crisps, sweets, ready meals, and fast food – stimulate your brain's reward circuits to abnormal levels, creating responses that easily overwhelm rational decision-making. This explains why certain foods can seem impossible to eat in moderation, even though you know about their impact. These foods aren't just enjoyable – they're engineered to trigger brain responses that can overwhelm rational control.

- **Constant Food Cues**: You're surrounded by reminders to eat – advertisements, visual displays, restaurants on every corner, apps that deliver food to your door – that automatically trigger eating responses. The sheer volume of these cues exceeds what you can effectively monitor and override through conscious thought. You feel this when you find yourself grabbing a snack while passing the kitchen, or reaching for extra food without thinking. These aren't conscious choices – they're automatic responses to environmental triggers, and there are more of these triggers than we've ever known before.

- **Social Eating Pressure**: You automatically tend to align your behavior with what seems normal in your environment. Exposure to situations where overeating is the norm creates powerful automatic drives to match those behaviors, regardless of your conscious knowledge about appropriate portions.

The Only Options Left

- You could become an even better expert on macronutrients, micronutrients, insulin response, and metabolic pathways, to make healthy choices automatic. But knowing that protein increases satiety doesn't help when you're emotionally eating ice cream at midnight. All the nutritional knowledge in the world can't override the behavioral patterns and emotional triggers that actually drive your eating when you haven't practised handling them.
- You could use detailed habit-tracking apps and productivity systems: perfect data and systematic tracking should create perfect behavior through increased awareness. But your history with dieting means any missed tick or imperfect day feels like failure. The pressure to maintain perfect streaks often leads to giving up entirely when you inevitably have an off day, and you conclude that you're too disorganized for any system to work.
- You could study the psychology of behavior change extensively: understanding the theory of willpower, motivation, and habit formation should make implementation automatic. But reading about behavior

change isn't the same as practising it. You can know all about habit-stacking and environmental design, but still struggle to actually form new eating habits because knowledge doesn't replace the repetitive practice needed to create automatic behavior.

- You could get continuous glucose monitors to track your body's responses: understanding how foods affect your energy levels should drive perfect food choices through data tracking. But then you'll become obsessed with keeping the numbers 'perfect', and normal energy fluctuations from healthy foods will trigger anxiety and restriction. The constant data stream will become another way to try 'thinking your way out' of problems that require behavioral practice, not more information.
- You could research every successful person's routine and try to copy them exactly: analysing what thin people eat and when they exercise should provide a proven blueprint for success. But their routines work for their genetics, lifestyle, and preferences – not yours. You can't copy and paste someone else's habits without doing the gradual work of building your own sustainable behaviors through trial and error and finding what actually works for your life.
- You could obsess over finding the 'perfect' meal timing and food combinations: researching circadian rhythm eating, food combining theories, and optimal meal timing should create the ideal eating schedule. But you're still trying to think your way into better

eating instead of practising the actual skills of eating according to your hunger, schedule, and preferences. Perfect timing means nothing if you haven't learned how to eat a satisfying meal without overeating.
- You could master every productivity method for food planning: learning elaborate meal prep systems, batch-cooking methods, and kitchen organization should make healthy eating effortless. But you're focused on finding the perfect system instead of building the actual skills of flexible meal planning. When your elaborate system inevitably breaks down due to life circumstances, you feel helpless because you've relied on the system instead of developing adaptive eating skills.

What You Actually Need

What you truly need is an approach that works with your brain's decision-making function rather than against it.

You need to understand that following through on what you know isn't about character. Recognizing that the gap between knowledge and action results from predictable neurological processes rather than personal weakness eliminates the secondary shame that makes implementation even harder.

You need environment modification rather than willpower enhancement. Creating physical and social environments that support rather than undermine your intentions dramatically reduces the cognitive burden of implementation. This isn't cheating – it's setting up your environment to work *with* the way your brain actually works.

You need systems that minimize how many decisions you have to make. Developing routines, habits, and predictable choices that reduce this number of decisions allows your limited mental energy to last longer before depletion triggers automatic processing.

Most importantly, you need to recognize that becoming successful isn't about becoming a different person with supernatural willpower. It's about creating conditions where your existing brain can function effectively despite its evolutionary limitations. There need to be systems in place around you, where what you know becomes what you naturally do, with minimal brain-strain. You have to assume that your motivation will waver and that being thin will not teach you impulse control.

You need to know how many steps away you are at any given time from turning a bad idea into a regrettable choice, the same way an addict in recovery must retain the humility to know they are only a couple of steps away from relapse if they do not create conditions that allow them to make calm, wise choices and remember their power. You too will need to keep an eye on your anxiety and stress levels, boredom and fatigue, knowing that your Achilles heel is extremes around food. This explains why willpower-based diets fail – you're asking System 2 to override System 1 indefinitely while restricting its fuel source. The framework in Part 3 works differently: it trains System 1 gradually so you're not constantly fighting your automatic responses.

Chapter 10

Joining the Dots: Why Understanding These Patterns Changes Everything

You may have been nodding along to some, or all, of these chapters thinking: *How does this person know exactly what's happening in my kitchen at midnight?* Or: *Is there a hidden camera in my car?* If so, you are starting to see what you've been struggling with all this time. What seemed like random failures or character flaws are in fact predictable, interconnected responses to the conditions created by repeated dieting:

- That loss of control when you start eating certain foods
- The constant food thoughts that won't quiet down
- The impossibility of moderation around trigger foods
- The overwhelming confusion about what to eat
- The automatic reliance on food when emotions rise
- The inability to keep certain foods in your house

- The self-sabotage just when success seems within reach
- The progressive weight gain despite countless diet attempts
- The gap between what you know and what you actually do

These seemingly separate struggles are connected pieces of the same puzzle – different ways in which your body and brain respond exactly as they're designed to when faced with perceived famine. These behaviors aren't happening because you're weak, undisciplined, or emotionally damaged. They're happening because you've been dieting. Each of these patterns is a direct, predictable result of food restriction. The very diets that promised to solve your weight problem have, over time, been creating and strengthening the exact behaviors that make lasting weight loss impossible. And these are the exact behaviors that push you from being that 'Too Much of a Good Thing' dieter to a Sensible Sobriety Seeker with a turbocharged eating disorder.

Of course, at this point you might be thinking: *I don't care about having an eating disorder – I just want to lose this weight!* I get it. Completely. And I'm not here to slap a label on you and tell you to give up on weight loss and focus solely on your mental health. I'm pointing this out because it's the missing piece that explains why you – a smart, accomplished person who can excel at pretty much anything else – haven't been able to 'crack the code' on weight loss.

It's not because you haven't found the right diet yet.

HOW DIETS MAKE US FAT

It's because dieting itself is creating the behaviors that guarantee your struggle. And because diet culture's pervasive influence leads people to believe from a young age that their worth is tied to being thin, and when they inevitably struggle to meet this goal, they feel inadequate and blame themselves for the flawed system. This sense of failure keeps them returning to endless products and programmes, creating a cycle of dependency (a very lucrative cycle for the diet industry).

When I am contacted by people who want help, it's always clear to me whether they've identified themselves as having an eating disorder. The language they use reveals their understanding of dieting's role in their struggle.

Two types of Sensible Sobriety Seekers

In my practice I see two types of Sensible Sobriety Seekers . . .

- **Type 1: Those Who Don't Recognize the Disorder**: People who don't consider themselves to have an eating disorder brought about by dieting blame themselves entirely for their current behaviors. They tell identical stories – repeated diets, mothers always on diets, hating their bodies, and a desperate desire to be free of thinking about food – but they frame it entirely as personal failing. They tend to have no time for examining what's gone before, insisting on taking full accountability even if they started dieting at 10 years old.
- **Type 2: Those Who Recognize the Disorder**: These are the people who *are* aware. They know that

dieting has given them an eating disorder; they also realize that their binge-restrict patterns are no different from those of someone with anorexia or bulimia. Put simply, the practical difference is that they binge more than they restrict and it shows up on their bodies as extra weight. They've been switching between restricting and bingeing since they were thin and have become stuck in this pattern. This is because it was initially effective at keeping them thin when their periods of restriction exceeded those of bingeing.

Even if a person does recognize the disorder, the Sensible Sobriety Seeker pattern is still largely invisible when it comes to research, treatment, and even conversations around eating and weight. The experience of the Sensible Sobriety Seeker has fallen through the cracks for several reasons. The first is that Sensible Sobriety Seeking often meets the criteria for multiple conditions that, in the past and currently, haven't been seen as interconnected problems or been addressed together.

Current diagnoses

Currently the actual diagnoses that explain what you've been experiencing fall into the following categories:
- **Yo-Yo Dieting**: The repeated cycle of losing and regaining weight, driven by strict dieting followed by reactive overeating
- **Weight Cycling**: The pattern of repeated weight

loss and regain, typically resulting from periods of restriction followed by inevitable rebound
- **Overshooting**: When weight regain after dieting exceeds your original starting weight, often due to both metabolic and psychological factors
- **Chronic Dieting**: Continuously engaging in dieting behaviors over years with little sustainable success, often switching between different approaches
- **Binge Eating Disorder**: Recurring episodes of eating large quantities of food rapidly to the point of discomfort, accompanied by feelings of guilt or distress
- **Compulsive Eating**: An uncontrollable urge to eat, often rapidly and to excess, typically triggered by emotional factors or food restriction
- **Emotional Eating**: Consuming food in response to emotional distress rather than physical hunger, using food to block negative feelings
- **Loss of Control Eating**: Feeling unable to stop eating once you've started, regardless of actual hunger or satiety signals
- **Food Addiction**: A behavioral addiction characterized by compulsive consumption of certain foods despite negative consequences

Yet, whether they blame themselves or not, what every one of my clients has realized is that their inability to maintain weight loss comes down to powerlessness around food. For many, this powerlessness extends beyond eating – it's a way of coping with difficult emotions like anger, unresolved pain, or overwhelming stress. However, diet culture frames the solution entirely through body size: *I'd be happy if I was thin*, rather than addressing the underlying issue, *I'd be happy if I felt in control of my choices*. I'm going to talk more about how diet culture has pushed this mindset in Part 2, but the effect has been that Sensible Sobriety Seekers have fallen between these diagnostic categories.

Why You're Invisible: The Diagnostic Gap

There are several reasons why Sensible Sobriety Seekers don't neatly fit the defined diagnostic categories. As I mentioned in Chapter 3, they don't meet the low weight criteria for anorexia, despite having almost identical psychological patterns of restriction and control. They may meet the criteria for Binge Eating Disorder, but treatment approaches for BED often fail to address their history of restriction and their continued attempts at extreme dieting. Traditional approaches to obesity may also completely miss the disordered eating patterns driving their weight gain.

Moreover, they often don't seek treatment for their disordered eating, specifically because they view their problem as a weight problem, rather than an eating disorder. This removes them from eating disorder statistics.

Their invisibility creates a cruel irony. The people most damaged by dieting – those caught in the most extreme cycles of restriction and binge – are exactly the ones most aggressively prescribed more dieting as the solution to their problems. It's like treating an alcoholic with a shot of vodka and then blaming them when they can't stop at one.

The Self-Reporting Problem

Sensible Sobriety Seekers also fall through a statistical gap. Studies on dieting and eating behaviors often rely on self-reported data, which is notoriously unreliable with Sensible Sobriety Seekers for several reasons. When asked, 'Are you currently dieting?' many Sensible Sobriety Seekers will say 'No,' even when they are planning to start a new diet the next day. They are perpetually between attempts, rather than actively dieting, which makes them fall off the radar in studies of dieters.

Sensible Sobriety Seekers also often severely under-report their food intake during binge periods due to shame, memory issues at times when they feel disconnected from what they are doing, or genuine uncertainty about what they've consumed. This results in apparently contradictory data: people who report eating less than their weight suggests and yet continue gaining. The yes/no nature of most diet research ('Are you on a diet?' Yes/No) completely misses the complex reality of someone who restricts periodically, binges reactively, and cycles between these two states, sometimes within a single day.

The Study Design Problem

Many diet studies have short timeframes (weeks to months) that can't capture the long-term pattern of restriction, followed by rebound weight gain, that defines the Sensible Sobriety Seekers experience. Dieting researchers typically exclude people with histories of eating disorders, yet include people with undiagnosed disordered eating – creating a selection bias that misses the very people most affected by dieting. Few studies follow the same individuals through multiple diet attempts over decades. This means they miss out on the long-term perspective needed to document the progressive intensification of the restriction-binge cycle that characterizes the Sensible Sobriety Seeker's journey.

The Dropout Factor

Even when Sensible Sobriety Seekers do participate in diet studies, they're more likely to drop out when restriction triggers binge episodes. Dropouts are typically excluded from final analyses, creating survivorship bias – where studies only show results from people who completed the programme, and hide the experiences of those who struggled most. This bias conceals the very pattern that defines this group.

Statistical invisibility creates a dangerous cycle: because Sensible Sobriety Seekers don't appear in research, research doesn't develop approaches that work for them. Because effective approaches aren't developed, Sensible Sobriety Seekers continue to struggle. And because they mainly struggle in isolation, they blame themselves, rather than recognizing that their experience is part of a widespread pattern that deserves scientific attention.

Understanding these patterns is the first step, but it raises a deeper question: why do some people develop these devastating patterns while others can diet occasionally without major drama? Why do some people spiral into Sensible Sobriety Seeking while others try a diet, abandon it, and move on with their lives? The answer lies in understanding the invisible forces that make certain people vulnerable to this cycle – and how modern conditions have amplified this vulnerability. Your individual struggle is part of a much larger story, one that reveals how systematic forces have created the perfect storm for Sensible Sobriety Seeking to flourish. To truly break free, you need to see not just your personal patterns, but the bigger picture that created them.

PART 2
THE BIGGER PICTURE

Chapter 11

Shame: The Invisible Accelerant

You've seen how Sensible Sobriety Seeking works: that desperate cycle of restriction, followed by the inevitable biological rebound that leads to gaining more weight despite trying harder than ever. But understanding this cycle isn't enough. We need to dig deeper into what makes it so stubbornly resistant to logic, willpower, and even the most determined efforts. The missing piece of this puzzle? Shame.

This is not just casual disappointment you feel when the scale doesn't budge or the frustration you experience when progress feels slow. As I said earlier, this is bone-deep identity-level shame that transforms something as basic as eating into a moral battleground. This isn't just one factor among many – it's the driving force behind why some people spiral down the Sensible Sobriety Seeker path at devastating speed while others can diet occasionally with minimal drama.

Consider two people attempting the same diet:

- **Person A has no history of body shame:** They approach weight loss as a practical matter. Perhaps their doctor suggested losing a few pounds for health reasons. When they feel hungry on their diet, they experience it as a physical sensation, perhaps uncomfortable but not emotionally charged. If they 'cheat' on their diet, they might feel mild disappointment but not profound self-loathing.
- **Person B has internalized deep shame about their body since childhood:** They approach weight loss as moral redemption – a way to finally become 'good enough'. When they feel hungry, they experience it as evidence of their greed and lack of discipline. If they 'cheat' on their diet, they experience devastating shame and self-hatred, often leading to dissociation and abandonment of all control.

Both experience the same biological drive to eat when restricting. However, Person A can approach this drive rationally, perhaps adjusting their plan to be more sustainable. Conversely, Person B experiences this drive as a personal failure that confirms their deepest fears about themselves, triggering the emotional overwhelm that leads to bingeing.

When Identity and Eating Collide: Shame Versus Guilt

Shame and guilt might sound like two words for the same feeling, but they create wildly different relationships with food. Guilt says: *I did something that didn't help my goals.* Shame declares: *I am fundamentally flawed because I ate.* This distinction isn't just psychological hairsplitting. It predicts your entire journey with food.

When you experience guilt about eating, you recognize a behavior that doesn't serve your goals while keeping your sense of worth intact. You might think: *I had more dessert than planned. Not ideal, but I'll adjust at my next meal.* That way the path ahead stays clear.

Shame, however, launches a full-scale assault on your core identity: *I ate dessert. I'm disgusting. I have no control. I'm a failure who will always be fat. What's the point?* This catastrophic dive doesn't just make you feel bad, it triggers a neurobiological cascade that makes balanced eating much harder. The person feeling guilt can simply course-correct. The person drowning in shame can only escape, either through the temporary high of extreme restriction or the momentary relief of bingeing until they can't feel anything. Neither provides any real solution, and they both only lead to increasingly severe cycles.

In my practice, I've noticed something fascinating: Sensible Sobriety Seekers often can't tell the difference between guilt and shame. When asked to describe how they differ, they look confused, because for them there is no separation. Every eating 'mistake' acts as further evidence that they're fundamentally defective as a human being. And this reveals a profound truth about their history. For Sensible Sobriety Seekers, shame wasn't something that became attached to eating later in life – it was their entry point to the entire world of food and their understanding of their bodies. Their earliest experiences with eating were already tainted by messages that their appetites were problematic, their bodies unacceptable, and their very desires somehow wrong.

The Shame-Addiction Connection: The Missing Link

Here's the game-changing insight that traditional weight management completely misses: if you want to predict who will develop Sensible Sobriety Seeking, look for people who are vulnerable to addiction. This is because the factors that create addiction vulnerability mirror those that create vulnerability to Sensible Sobriety Seeking. This isn't just a coincidence: it's causation.

Your brain processes shame and physical pain through overlapping neural pathways – both activate similar distress signals and trigger urgent needs for relief. So shame actually rewires your brain's reward and regulation systems in ways that create addiction-like patterns with both restriction and food.

For the shame-vulnerable person, both restriction and bingeing can become powerful relief mechanisms: restriction provides temporary escape through the feeling of virtuousness and control, creating a brain reward that becomes addictively reinforcing despite being ultimately destructive. When biology inevitably kicks in, bingeing creates relief through dissociation: a detachment from self-awareness that temporarily numbs the unbearable shame.

With each cycle, these patterns become more entrenched, more extreme, and more resistant to rational intervention, exactly as we see in addiction.

This explains why willpower-based approaches are so spectacularly unsuccessful for Sensible Sobriety Seekers. You're not facing a simple behavior choice. You're battling powerful neurochemical forces in your brain created by shame.

Your Brain and Shame: The Neurological Ambush

When shame enters the picture, it doesn't just make you feel bad; it transforms your brain function in ways that make sensible eating neurologically impossible. Here's how: the brain's executive function centre – responsible for planning, decision-making, and impulse control – becomes dramatically impaired during states of shame. It can cause activity in the prefrontal cortex, creating conditions where balanced, moderate choices become impossible. This isn't weakness or lack of discipline. It's your neurobiology responding exactly as it's designed to when you find yourself under threat.

Intense shame triggers dissociation, a protective psychological state where you disconnect from your current experience. This explains why you might not remember eating an entire packet of biscuits or you might feel as if you were taken over by someone else. Your brain is protecting you from shame so overwhelming it feels as if it could destroy your core self. Shame creates such intense psychological pain that your brain prioritizes immediate relief above all else. For Sensible Sobriety Seekers, food, particularly highly palatable food, becomes the fastest accessible path to numbing this pain. The urge to binge isn't about hunger or enjoyment; it's about escaping psychological anguish.

Shame also creates all-or-nothing thinking where only perfect adherence feels acceptable. This explains why a single biscuit can trigger complete abandonment of your eating plan. Your brain isn't evaluating the nutritional impact; it's responding to the catastrophic message that you've failed as a person.

And, perhaps most insidiously, shame actively disrupts memory formation and retrieval, creating a type of amnesia that prevents you from recognizing harmful patterns in your eating. This is why you can have the same 'last binge' hundreds of times without seeing an obvious cycle. Your brain is actually preventing the formation of connections that would make the pattern visible. These neurobiological effects create perfect conditions for Sensible Sobriety Seeking to develop and intensify.

The Earliest Wound: Shame Before Choice

For most Sensible Sobriety Seekers , shame wasn't something that developed after weight gain or failed diets; it was established early, often before they had any conscious control over their eating or body size.

Some lucky kids grow up experiencing food primarily as nourishment: eating feels neutral, even pleasurable. Their earliest relationship with food builds a foundation of trust that hunger is valid, fullness deserves respect, and eating is as natural as breathing. But others experience a profoundly different initiation. Maybe you were that child who noticed you were getting smaller portions than your siblings, as if your hunger was somehow less legitimate? Perhaps you heard adults discussing your body with concern or disapproval before you even understood what weight management meant?

Some children were put on special diets while other family members ate 'normally', absorbing the message that their body was defective and others were acceptable? If you're a woman, you might have watched your mother obsessively controlling her own eating while praising thinness. Maybe this taught you that female worth is tied to body size long before you could question this belief? Or perhaps you were teased about your size at school while adults did nothing, teaching you that body shame was socially acceptable?

Many Sensible Sobriety Seekers report learning early that being 'good', while satisfying, was shameful. This early imprinting doesn't just teach you that certain foods are 'bad'. It teaches you that you are bad for wanting them. It doesn't just suggest that weight gain is undesirable. It implies that your body itself is unacceptable. This creates a fundamental fracture in your relationship with food and your body that conventional approaches completely miss.

The child with this early stamp of shame develops a profoundly different relationship with food from the child who only encountered diet messages later in life. Where others might experience dieting as a temporary behavior change, the shame-imprinted child experiences it as an identity project: a desperate attempt to finally become acceptable after years of feeling fundamentally flawed.

The Cruel Paradox: How Desperation Drives Weight Gain

The most painful irony of Sensible Sobriety Seeking is that the people most desperate to lose weight – those with the highest levels of body shame – are precisely the ones most likely to experience progressive weight gain.

This isn't coincidence or lack of effort – it's the predictable outcome of the way shame transforms eating behavior. More shame creates more extreme restriction. When your very worth feels tied to your size, moderate approaches feel woefully inadequate. Only dramatic, often dangerous measures feel proportionate to the existential importance of weight loss. So you are not choosing extreme diets because you are ignorant. You're choosing them because they match the intensity of your shame.

This extreme restriction triggers a powerful biological backlash. Your body responds to severe calorie reduction as the survival emergency it is, activating multiple systems to restore energy balance. The more extreme your restriction, the more powerful this response. When this inevitable compensation occurs, shame intensifies to catastrophic levels. Rather than recognizing this as a normal physiological response, you experience it as confirmation of your worthlessness. The shame is so unbearable that it triggers dissociation and memory disruption, preventing you from learning from the experience.

This intensified shame drives even more extreme restriction attempts. To compensate for what feels like a profound moral failure, you pursue increasingly desperate measures, creating an even more severe biological emergency. What started as 'eating healthier' escalates to eliminating food groups, then skipping meals, then fasting – each attempt more extreme because the shame demands it. With each cycle, the pattern becomes more severe and the weight gain more significant. What might be a five-pound fluctuation in someone with low shame becomes a 50-pound gain in someone with high shame: not because they care less about their weight but because they care so much that it drives approaches guaranteed to backfire.

Longitudinal research reveals a paradox: greater weight preoccupation predicts worse long-term weight outcomes. The more intensely you pursue thinness through restriction, the more powerful the biological and psychological backlash.

Modern Conditions: The Perfect Shame Storm

Today's environment has created a perfect storm of factors that maximize shame while simultaneously making its consequences more severe. We live in a culture that connects fundamental worth to thinness while surrounding us with idealized images designed to make even healthy bodies feel inadequate. And social media creates unprecedented

HOW DIETS MAKE US FAT

opportunities for us to compare our appearance, exposing us to curated images that continually activate shame.

At the same time, we navigate a food environment engineered to override natural regulation, with products designed by teams of scientists to maximize consumption by targeting addiction pathways in the brain. Ultra-processed food, in particular, targets the exact neurobiological vulnerabilities created by shame.

Then, through the diet industry, we're encouraged to attempt weight loss using approaches that trigger biological starvation responses, despite the long-term weight-loss data being consistent – the vast majority of dieters regain weight. If you've regained, you're not the exception. You're the rule. The wellness industry has simply rebranded restriction as 'clean eating' or 'lifestyle change', making the shame component more powerful by adding moral virtue to any concerns over a person's appearance. And the recent emergence of weight-loss medications such as Ozempic and Wegovy has added another layer to this perfect shame storm, promising pharmaceutical solutions while reinforcing the message that your natural body is a medical problem requiring intervention.

Eventually, when our bodies respond exactly as they're designed to in response to such impossible conditions, we're taught to blame ourselves rather than question the approach. And for people with a predisposition towards shame, these conditions guarantee progressive weight gain. It's like forcing someone to hold their breath underwater, blaming them when they eventually gasp for air, and then claiming their 'lack of breathing control' is the problem.

Today's stressful lifestyles also deplete the exact neurological resources needed for moderation and self-regulation, creating conditions where even people who previously had healthy relationships with food become vulnerable to shame-driven patterns. And it is these modern conditions that help explain why obesity rates have risen dramatically, despite the unprecedented focus on weight loss. It's not because people have suddenly become lazy or undisciplined; it's because we've created the exact conditions that maximize the expression of Sensible Sobriety Seeking in vulnerable individuals.

The Revelation That Changes Everything

Understanding shame's role in Sensible Sobriety Seeking reveals some-thing even more profound. This condition didn't develop by accident. The shame that drives Sensible Sobriety Seeking was established and continuously reinforced by a system designed to keep you trapped. And some people are far more vulnerable to this shame-based manipulation than others.

When you recognize that your 'personal failure' is actually a predictable response to conditions specifically designed to exploit certain vulnerabilities, everything changes. The path to freedom begins with seeing the cage that's been built around you, and recognizing that you have the power to dismantle it, one shame-free choice at a time.

Chapter 12
Why Some People Get Trapped Faster

I've seen countless accelerated paths leading to 'Restriction Addiction'. Growing up in food-insecure households where scarcity taught you to eat whenever food appeared. Experiencing prolonged stress where a particular food became your primary coping mechanism. Being praised for weight loss then shamed when biology forced regain. Learning that food could soothe overwhelming emotional pain, then being blamed for the resulting weight gain.

I'm focusing on ADHD, autism, and trauma because these are the patterns I see most frequently in my practise and they reveal the clearest mechanistic links to Restriction Addiction. ADHD affects dopamine regulation and impulse control, the exact systems restriction disrupts further. Autism often involves sensory sensitivities and need for routine making the rigid structure of restriction feel safer than the chaos of flexible eating. Trauma dysregulates the nervous system and emotional processing, creating conditions where food becomes a primary tool for managing unbearable internal states.

Understanding these connections explains why standard advice – 'just eat normally', 'practice moderation', 'trust your body' – fails so catastrophically for people with these traits. The framework works regardless of whether you have ADHD, autism, trauma, or perfectionist patterns. But if you do, understanding the specific interaction between your traits and restriction behavior makes the work exponentially more effective. I didn't realize it when I was writing my earlier books, but certain conditions profoundly influenced my relationship with food. This isn't about excusing the behaviors but understanding the neurobiological foundation that makes some people significantly more vulnerable to food obsession, diet culture, and Sensible Sobriety Seeking.

I was diagnosed with Attention Deficit Hyperactivity Disorder (ADHD) in my late thirties, long after I'd developed the patterns we've been discussing. Looking back, it explained so much about why conventional approaches had felt impossible for me while seemingly working for others. But it wasn't until I started hearing thousands of stories that I began to see the same pattern emerging again and again: certain neurological differences and life experiences created a perfect storm of vulnerability to the shame-based manipulation of diet culture.

The research on this connection is still limited, but an increasing body of evidence is identifying clear links between neurodevelopmental differences, trauma histories, and eating disorders. What I've observed in my practice goes far beyond what the studies capture – I've seen how these vulnerabilities interact with modern diet culture to create the exact conditions for Sensible Sobriety Seeking to flourish.

If you have been diagnosed with ADHD like me, or you suspect you could be, or you relate to traits exhibited by neurodivergent people, then this system can be particularly devastating. If you've experienced trauma, if you're naturally a perfectionist, or if you have other neurological differences, diet culture doesn't just fail you – it actively exploits the very wiring that makes you unique. Understanding why can finally help you stop blaming yourself for struggling with approaches that were never designed for your brain.

When Your Brain Works Differently

Research documents significant associations between ADHD and disordered eating patterns, with elevated rates of binge-eating disorder among ADHD populations. People with ADHD may experience differences in dopamine signalling, reward response, and impulse control, which can make rigid rules more difficult to follow consistently . . .

- **Lower baseline dopamine levels** can make you more sensitive to reward and more likely to seek intense experiences. When diet culture promises dramatic transformation and quick results, your ADHD brain finds this irresistible in a way that steady, moderate approaches simply can't match.
- **Stronger reward-seeking behaviors** can make forbidden foods more attractive. The more something is

restricted, the more your brain fixates on it. This isn't poor impulse control – it's how ADHD brains are wired to respond to limitations.
- **More intense reactions to both restriction and reward** can intensify the cycle. When you restrict, the deprivation feels more unbearable. When you finally eat forbidden foods, the experience of relief and pleasure can feel more intense, which may reinforce patterns of restrictive eating and bingeing.
- **Greater difficulty with impulse control** can make resisting cravings harder, especially when those cravings have been intensified by restriction. What looks like weakness is actually a neurological reality.
- **Executive function challenges** can make complex food rules almost impossible to follow consistently. Meal planning, tracking, and constant decision-making about food exhaust your limited executive function resources faster than they would for neurotypical people.

When you restrict food, dopamine levels drop further, creating even more intense cravings and reward-seeking behaviors. This isn't moral weakness; it's simply that ADHD can make consistent adherence to restrictive plans more difficult, which some people experience as intense cycles of restriction and overeating.

The diet industry doesn't acknowledge this vulnerability – in fact, it exploits it. Marketing often targets those who struggle most with impulse control and emotional regulation, promising simple solutions without acknowledging the neurobiological factors that make these solutions particularly challenging for certain brains.

For some people with ADHD, shame creates an even more powerful vulnerability to the Sensible Sobriety Seeking pattern. The ADHD brain struggles to consistently control certain impulses, and finds delayed gratification and sustained attention more difficult – the very skills conventional weight-loss approaches demand. When shame enters the equation, it dramatically amplifies these challenges.

Sometimes, when someone with ADHD tries to follow a 'sensible' eating plan, their decision-making capacity is already compromised. Dopamine differences can create stronger-than-average cravings for high-reward foods. Their time perception can make delayed rewards (future weight loss) less motivating than immediate ones (the pleasure of eating). Now add shame to this reality. When they inevitably struggle with an approach that was never designed for their brain type, they don't attribute it to a mismatch between the method and their neurology. Instead, the shame narrative tells them they're lazy, undisciplined, or broken. This shame triggers more impulsivity, stronger cravings, and further executive function impairment – creating a vicious cycle.

The Autism Connection: When Structure Traps You

The same need for structure that some autistic people rely on can become a trap when those rules inevitably prove unsustainable...

- **Sensory processing differences** can make certain foods overwhelming while others provide comfort. Diet culture's demonization of comfort foods can remove your primary sensory regulation tools, creating distress that manifests as eating difficulties.
- **All-or-nothing thinking patterns** make the diet culture's 'good food/bad food' messaging particularly powerful. Where others might see flexibility, some autistic people see clear categories that must be followed perfectly. This creates the same all-or-nothing patterns we see in Sensible Sobriety Seeking.
- **Routine disruption sensitivity** means that when a diet plan becomes unsustainable, the entire eating structure can collapse. Unlike neurotypical people who might adjust gradually, autistic people often experience complete system breakdown when their food rules stop working.
- **Social communication differences** can make it harder to seek help or communicate struggles with eating. The shame around 'failing' at diets can be particularly intense when you've been masking other differences your whole life.
- **Intense special interests** can become focused on food, nutrition, or weight loss, creating an obsessive quality that goes far beyond typical dieting. What starts as an interest in health can become an all-consuming preoccupation that dominates daily life. The intersection of autism and diet culture creates the perfect conditions for Sensible Sobriety Seeking

because the promise of clear rules appeals to some autistic people, but the biological reality of those rules creates impossible contradictions that the autistic nervous system struggles to resolve.

The Trauma Connection: When Past Meets Present

People with histories of trauma also have a unique vulnerability to the Sensible Sobriety Seeking pattern. Trauma, particularly early developmental trauma, creates lasting changes in how the nervous system processes threat, safety, and bodily sensations.

For trauma survivors, restriction can initially provide a false sense of control in a world that once felt dangerously out of control. The clarity of rigid food rules can temporarily soothe the hyper-vigilance common in people who have experienced trauma. But this relief is short-lived . . .

- **Hyper-vigilance in the nervous system** means that when restriction triggers physical hunger, your traumatized nervous system may interpret this as a survival threat, activating the fight-flight-freeze responses. In this activated state, the prefrontal cortex (responsible for decision-making) goes offline while the amygdala (emotional alarm system) takes control. This makes reasoned choices around food almost impossible, creating what feels like 'out of control' eating but is actually a predictable trauma response.

- **Disconnection from body signals** often develops as a protective mechanism during trauma. If your body wasn't safe during traumatic experiences, you learned to disconnect from its signals. This makes intuitive eating approaches particularly challenging because the signals you're supposed to trust were once associated with danger.
- **Emotional dysregulation** means that everyday difficult feelings can become more overwhelming more quickly. Food becomes one of the few available tools for managing intense emotions, especially when other coping mechanisms feel too vulnerable or aren't readily accessible. **Trust issues extend to trusting your own body and its needs.** When you've been hurt by people who were supposed to protect you, learning to trust your body's hunger and fullness signals can feel equally dangerous. As restriction triggers the biological compensation mechanisms we've discussed, the resulting intensity of hunger signals can mimic the physiological arousal of trauma. The body doesn't distinguish between types of distress – it simply registers threat. This creates a devastating cycle where restriction triggers trauma responses, which then trigger bingeing as an attempt to regulate the nervous system, which creates shame, which reinforces the need for control through restriction. This trauma-restriction cycle helps explain why seemingly minor disruptions can trigger major binges in Sensible Sobriety Seekers. What looks like 'lack of willpower' is actually a

profoundly dysregulated nervous system desperately seeking safety in the only way it knows how.

The Perfectionist: All-or-Nothing Thinking

If you tend towards perfectionism, the all-or-nothing thinking of diet culture also creates special vulnerability. Perfectionism often manifests as extreme rules that are impossible to maintain. When these rules are inevitably broken, the perfectionist doesn't adjust – they abandon. This creates the 'what-the-hell effect' where one deviation leads to complete collapse . . .

- **Impossibly high standards** mean that anything less than perfect adherence feels like complete failure. A perfectionist can't just have one biscuit and move on – they've either followed the rules perfectly or they've failed completely.
- **Fear of making mistakes** can make eating feel like a constant test. Every food choice becomes an opportunity to either succeed or fail at being 'good', creating enormous pressure around basic nourishment.
- **Identity tied to achievement** means that diet 'failure' isn't just disappointing – it threatens a core sense of self. When your worth is tied to success, diet struggles feel like evidence of fundamental inadequacy.
- **Difficulty with flexibility** makes moderate approaches feel unsafe. For perfectionists, moderation can feel more threatening than restriction because it lacks

clear boundaries. Without definitive rules about what's 'allowed', eating becomes anxiety-provoking rather than satisfying.

The diet industry specifically exploits perfectionism, promising clear rules and definitive 'success' metrics that appeal to the perfectionist mindset while guaranteeing eventual failure. The language of diet culture – 'clean eating', 'cheat days', 'good foods' versus 'bad foods' – speaks directly to perfectionist psychology while setting up impossible standards.

Why Conventional Approaches Fail These Brains

Understanding these vulnerabilities reveals why standard weight-loss advice fails so consistently for certain people. When someone with ADHD is told to 'just use moderation', they could be being asked to do something their brain isn't wired to do easily. When some people with autism are told to 'listen to their body', they may be more disconnected from subtle internal signals than others. When someone with trauma history is told to 'trust their hunger', they're being asked to trust a system that once failed to protect them.

The shame that follows these inevitable 'failures' isn't just disappointing – it can confirm these individuals' worst fears about themselves. The ADHD person thinks they have no self-control. The autistic person thinks they're too rigid. The trauma survivor thinks they're broken. The perfectionist thinks they're not good enough.

This shame drives more extreme attempts to succeed, creating exactly the conditions for Sensible Sobriety Seeking to develop. What starts as a desire to be healthier becomes a desperate attempt to prove worthiness through food control – a battle that these particular brains are neurologically destined to lose.

The Modern Amplification

Today's environment has again created the perfect conditions for these vulnerabilities to be expressed more intensely than ever before. The proliferation of conflicting diet information overwhelms executive function in those already struggling with decision-making. The ultra-processed food environment specifically targets the reward systems that are already dysregulated in these populations.

Most critically, the shame-based messaging of diet culture has become more sophisticated and pervasive. Where previous generations might have encountered occasional diet messaging, today's vulnerable individuals are surrounded by it constantly – through social media, wellness culture, and the medicalization of body size – where normal variations in body weight are increasingly classified as diseases requiring treatment. This explains why we're seeing rising rates of eating disorders across all these populations. It's not that more people are developing these neurological differences or trauma histories – it's that the environment has become increasingly toxic for those who have them.

The Missing Piece

Understanding your specific vulnerabilities isn't about making excuses or accepting limitations. It's about finally understanding why approaches that work for others have felt impossible for you. When you stop trying to force your unique brain to work like a neurotypical brain, when you stop blaming yourself for struggling with approaches that weren't designed for your wiring, you can finally start building strategies that actually work. Once you understand this, you can stop fighting your neurology and start working *with* it.

But first, you need to understand how this shame-based system has been deliberately constructed to keep you trapped – and how it operates exactly like an abusive relationship designed to make you believe you can't survive without it.

Chapter 13

The Abusive Relationship with Diet Culture

I want to show you why all those approaches you've tried – all those sensible plans, mindful strategies, and lifestyle changes – were doomed from the start. It's not because you lacked willpower. It's because you've been trapped in an abusive relationship with diet culture that has created addiction-like dependencies so powerful that conventional approaches never stood a chance. And like all abusive relationships, this one uses specific tactics to keep you trapped. Let me walk you through exactly how this relationship operates, and why it's left you feeling powerless around food.

Love-Bombing: The Seduction Phase

Every diet begins the same way – with intoxicating promises of transformation. This doesn't just focus on weight loss, but a complete reinvention of your life: 'This time will be different;' 'Your real life can finally begin;' 'Everything you want is on the other side of this weight loss;' 'You'll finally have the confidence you deserve;' 'You'll be the person you were always meant to be.'

Remember that rush of hope at the start of each new plan? The fantasy of how different life would be once you lost the weight? The belief that this time, finally, it would stick? That's love-bombing. An overwhelming flood of promises and excitement designed to create a powerful emotional attachment.

Then, there's the before-and-after photos; the emotional testimonials; the celebrity transformations; the scientific-sounding explanations that make this approach seem different from all the others. It's all designed to create a powerful emotional bond before the abuse cycle begins. And the more desperate you feel about your body, the more powerful this hook becomes. When you hate yourself in your current body, the promise of transformation takes on an almost religious significance. This isn't about vanity, it's about salvation.

You're not stupid for falling for this repeatedly. You're human, responding to one of the most powerful psychological manipulation tactics known.

Gaslighting: Destroying Your Trust in Your Body

After years in this relationship, you probably don't even know when you're truly hungry or full anymore. Diet culture has taught you to distrust your body's signals. It tells you untruths such as:

HOW DIETS MAKE US FAT

- 'You're not really hungry – you're just bored.'
- 'If you were truly listening to your body, you wouldn't want that food.'
- 'That feeling isn't real hunger – real hunger feels different.'
- 'Your cravings are just addiction – you need to break free from them.'
- 'Your body is lying to you – trust the plan instead.'
- 'Everyone else can manage moderation – what's wrong with you?'

But this is gaslighting. It's making you question your own reality, and it's a cornerstone of abuse. Diet culture undermines your ability to trust your most basic bodily signals, replacing your internal wisdom with external rules created by so-called experts who claim to know your body better than you do. When you feel hungry, you can't trust that feeling. When you enjoy a food item, you can't trust that pleasure.

This gaslighting extends beyond food. Diet culture teaches you to distrust your perception of your own body. When you look in the mirror, you can't trust what you see. After years of this, you become completely disconnected from your internal signals. No wonder 'intuitive eating' seems impossible – you've been trained to override intuition in favour of an arbitrary set of rules.

When a diet inevitably fails, the gaslighting intensifies: 'The plan works for everyone who follows it correctly. If it didn't work for you, you must have done something wrong.' Just like an abuse victim who begins to believe they're crazy or imagining things, you start to think your experience is uniquely flawed rather than evidence of a broken system.

Isolation: Cutting You Off From Support

Abusers systematically isolate their victims, cutting them off from supportive relationships and alternative perspectives. Diet culture isolates you on three critical levels . . .

- **Physical isolation:** You avoid social eating situations where you can't control the food offered to you. You decline invitations to parties with 'temptations'. You prepare and eat different foods than family or friends. You eat before dates so you won't have to eat 'normally' in public. You bring special food to gatherings or refuse to eat what everyone else is enjoying. You think the following thoughts: *I can't go to that restaurant – there's nothing on the menu that fits my plan; I'll skip the office birthday celebration – I don't need the temptation; I'll just have a salad while everyone else has pizza – I'm being 'good' today.* This physical separation reduces your opportunities to reality-test your experiences with others. When you're not participating in normal social eating, you can't see that most people eat a variety of foods without obsession or shame.
- **Internal isolation:** You learn to ignore or override your body's natural signals: hunger, fullness, satisfaction, pleasure. The wisdom of your body, evolved over millions of years to regulate weight naturally, gets

silenced in favour of external rules. You tell yourself: *I'm not supposed to be hungry yet – it's not time to eat; I shouldn't be full yet – I've only had half my portion; I shouldn't want that – it's a 'bad' food.* This internal disconnection leaves you unable to access your built-in guidance system. Like someone who's been taught to ignore the sensation of needing to use the bathroom, you eventually lose the ability to recognize the signal until it's at emergency levels.

- **Social isolation:** Most critically, the shame around diet failure prevents you from discussing your struggles openly. You hide binges, weight regain, and the emotional toll of dieting. You present a carefully curated version of your relationship with food to the world. You devise face-saving workarounds such as: *I'll tell everyone I'm not hungry rather than admit I'm on a diet; I'll hide the wrappers from my binge so no one knows; I'll pretend I'm making progress even when I'm struggling.*

This secrecy creates the illusion that you're uniquely broken while everyone else successfully maintains control. It prevents the collective realization that would threaten diet culture's power: that almost everyone is failing at dieting, for the same structural reasons. This isolation becomes self-reinforcing. The more ashamed you feel, the less you share. The less you share, the more alone you feel in your struggle. The more alone you feel, the more vulnerable you become to diet culture's next 'solution'.

SHAHROO IZADI

Intermittent Reinforcement: The Gambling Psychology of Dieting

Abusive relationships often involve 'intermittent reinforcement' – unpredictable patterns of reward and punishment that create powerful attachment. This is also precisely how diet culture operates.

The initial days of a diet often bring positive reinforcement: quick water weight loss (the initial pounds that drop rapidly, due to reduced glycogen stores and lower fluid retention), compliments from others, a sense of virtue and control. This early success keeps you believing in the system. Then comes the inevitable physiological pushback: your weight loss plateaus, hunger intensifies, the cravings become overwhelming. The diet system treats these normal biological responses as personal failures. Occasionally, through unhealthy extremes, you might experience brief 'successes'. Perhaps you reach your goal weight temporarily or fit into a smaller clothing size, before the biological compensation kicks in again, bringing punishment in the form of weight regain and shame.

This unpredictable pattern of reward and punishment doesn't weaken your attachment to dieting, it strengthens it. In fact, intermittent reinforcement creates the strongest behavioral conditioning. This is why gambling is so addictive: the occasional, unpredictable win keeps you playing, despite consistent losses. Each small, temporary success renews your hope that next time will be different, even as the overall pattern clearly shows it won't be. And, just like the gambler who remembers every win but discounts every loss, you remember each moment of dieting 'success' while explaining away the much longer periods of 'failure'. This selective memory isn't a character flaw – it's a psychological response to intermittent reinforcement, one of the most powerful conditioning tools available.

Moving the Goalposts: Ensuring You Can Never Win

Abusers maintain control by creating impossible standards that constantly shift, ensuring the victim can never succeed or feel secure. Diet culture has perfected this tactic. When you reach your initial goal weight, there's suddenly a new problem to fix. Now you need to tone up. Now you need more muscle definition. Now you need to lose those last five pounds. Now you need to maintain, which means continuing the same restrictive behaviors forever.

The messaging shifts from 'lose weight to be healthy' to 'lose weight to be attractive' to 'lose weight to prove your discipline' to 'lose weight because you've always been trying to lose weight.' The goal is never really a specific size or number – it's just a constant pursuit. Because as long as you're pursuing, you're consuming diet culture's products, programmes, and ideology.

These shifting goalposts ensure that you never reach a point of satisfaction or completion, exactly as an abuser wants their victim to feel. Just at the moment when you might feel successful and therefore independent, the definition of success changes, keeping you dependent on the system for validation you can never quite achieve.

Trauma Bonding: The Biochemical Addiction

In abusive relationships, trauma bonding – a psychological phenomenon where victims develop positive feelings towards their abuser through cycles of abuse and intermittent kindness – creates powerful attachment through alternating fear and relief. This cycle can create strong attachment patterns and reinforce habitual responses, sometimes resembling addiction-like neural pathways.

The restriction phase increases stress hormones like cortisol while creating dopamine anticipation of future reward (*I'll be so happy when I lose the weight*). The inevitable breaking point triggers a flood of relief chemicals – dopamine, serotonin, endorphins – as you finally eat forbidden foods.

This relief is immediately followed by intense shame, creating another cortisol spike that drives the need for more relief. You return to restriction as the only way to escape the shame, beginning the cycle again. The more times you cycle through restriction and bingeing, the more deeply these pathways get entrenched, making each subsequent attempt at control more likely to fail. This trauma bonding explains why simply knowing diets don't work isn't enough to break free. Your attachment isn't logical – it's biochemical. Just as an abuse victim may intellectually know they should leave but feel unable to do so, you may know dieting damages you while still feeling powerless to stop.

Learned Helplessness: When You Stop Believing Freedom is Possible

The ultimate goal of an abusive relationship is to create 'learned helplessness', the psychological state where victims stop believing escape is possible. Diet culture creates this state through repeated experiences of failure. After years of cycling through diets, many people reach a state of complete helplessness. They convince themselves: *I can't trust myself around food; I'll always struggle with my weight; I need external rules to function; I'll never have a 'normal' relationship with eating; this is just how I am – I have no willpower; I need someone else to tell me what to eat.*

This learned helplessness is the ultimate win for the diet industry. Once you believe you're fundamentally broken and incapable of eating without strict control, you become a lifelong customer, not because their products work, but because you can't imagine existing without them.

Even when, intellectually, you know diets don't work, even when you've experienced their failure firsthand dozens of times, this state of learned helplessness keeps you trapped in the cycle. You can't conceive of a way of eating that isn't either rigid control or complete chaos.

Identity Fusion: When Dieting Becomes Who You Are

The final stage of this abusive relationship is when dieting becomes fused with your identity. This happens when you've been dieting for so long that you don't know who you would be without it. You tell yourself: *I'm a person who's always trying to lose weight*; *I'm good when I'm on a diet and bad when I'm off it*; *my worth is tied to my ability to control my eating*; *I'm someone who struggles with food*.

This identity fusion explains why the idea of stopping dieting can feel like a kind of grief. You can't imagine who you would be without this defining struggle. Your entire adult life may have been structured around cycles of dieting, making the prospect of living without it both liberating and terrifying.

The Multiple Addictions Diet Culture Creates

But the abusive relationship with diet culture doesn't just create one addiction. It creates several interconnected dependencies that reinforce each other . . .

- **Addiction to Restriction: The Control High**: For some chronic dieters, restriction itself becomes addictive. The sense of control, virtue, and moral superiority from successfully following rigid food rules creates a powerful dopamine rush. This 'restriction high' can become so reinforced that you continue restricting even when you know it's harmful. You might experience anxiety when you can't follow your food rules; a sense of superiority when restricting; a rush of pleasure when successfully avoiding 'bad' foods; continued restriction despite the negative physical consequences; and a need for increasingly strict rules to feel 'in control'. This addiction explains why many people can't simply 'eat flexibly' even when they intellectually understand the harm of dieting. The psychological rewards of restriction have become too powerful to abandon.

- **Addiction to Sugar and Hyper-palatable Foods:** The restrict-binge cycle also directly heightens your neurological response to highly palatable foods, especially those combining sugar, fat, and salt. Restriction lowers dopamine and serotonin levels, creating a neurochemical state similar to withdrawal. When you finally eat the 'forbidden' foods, the reward response is intensified, creating a stronger association between these foods and relief. The cycle strengthens with each restriction-binge episode. What makes this particularly insidious is that the very foods diet culture demonize become increasingly powerful through the act of demonizing them.

- **Addiction to Emotional Eating:** The emotional relief that comes from eating after restriction can become a powerful coping mechanism. Restriction creates psychological distress and so eating forbidden foods provides temporary relief. This relief teaches your brain that food is an effective emotional regulator. Over time, you turn to food automatically when experiencing difficult emotions. This isn't a character flaw; it's a learned association reinforced by thousands of experiences where food was your only reliable source of comfort in a system designed to make you feel perpetually inadequate.

- **Addiction to the Diet Cycle Itself:** Perhaps most powerfully, many become addicted to the diet cycle as a whole: the dramatic ups and downs, the hope of transformation, the purging of shame through restriction. The anticipation of starting a new diet triggers dopamine release. The early success phase provides validation and excitement. Even the shame after failing can create a biochemical response. The relief of starting over completes the addictive cycle. This explains why many people continue cycling through diets for decades despite consistent failure. The cycle itself – restriction, hope, failure, shame, renewal – has become rewarding, even as it damages physical and psychological health.

Breaking Free From the Abuse

Understanding this abusive relationship is the first step towards freedom. When you recognize that your struggles aren't personal failures but predictable responses to manipulation, everything changes.

The multiple addictions this system creates can't be broken through willpower alone. They require specific strategies that address the neurobiological and psychological patterns that have been established. But before we explore those solutions, you need to understand why every other approach you've tried has failed – and why they were designed to fail people like you from the start.

Chapter 14

Why Nothing Else Has Worked

You've tried everything. You've followed the meal plans, tracked the macros, practised mindful eating, attempted intuitive eating, joined support groups, and worked with therapists. You've read books about body acceptance and health at every size. You've tried the moderate approaches and the extreme ones. You've attempted to just 'eat sensibly' and 'use portion control'. And none of it has stuck.

This isn't because you're broken, undisciplined, or haven't found the right approach yet. It's because every one of these methods fails to address your complete set of needs. You're not dealing with a simple weight problem or even a straightforward eating disorder. You're dealing with the neurobiological aftermath of abuse that has created multiple addiction-like dependencies. And none of the conventional approaches are designed to deal with that reality.

What You Actually Need

Before we examine why everything has failed, let's be clear about what you really need – the complete package that would finally work:

- **Weight loss that you can actually keep off**: Not through unsustainable restriction, but by healing the patterns that drive weight regain. You want to lose weight and maintain it without constantly fearing that it will all come back (plus more).
- **A sense of personal power around food:** The ability to make calm, confident decisions about eating without feeling controlled by cravings, emotions, or external rules. You want to feel as if you're in charge of your choices rather than food being in charge of you.
- **Freedom from food obsession:** The mental space that comes when food stops dominating your thoughts. You want to be able to think about other things, to have conversations that aren't about dieting, to live a life where food is just one aspect rather than the central drama.
- **The ability to enjoy food again:** To experience pleasure in eating without guilt, shame, or fear. You want to be able to celebrate with food, to enjoy meals with others, to taste and savour without constant moral judgment.
- **Comfort from food when you need it:** The capacity to use food for emotional comfort occasionally

without it spiralling into destructive patterns. You want food to be available as one tool for comfort among many, not your only or primary coping mechanism.

- **A body you can accept:** Not necessarily love every minute, but one you can inhabit comfortably, appreciate for its capabilities, and treat with basic kindness regardless of its size.
- **Freedom from shame:** The ability to eat imperfectly without catastrophic self-loathing. You want to be able to make mistakes around food and move on without it confirming deep beliefs about your worth as a person.
- **Skills that transfer to other areas:** Confidence, self-regulation, and decision-making abilities that improve your entire life, not just your eating. You want the process of healing your relationship with food to make you stronger and more capable in all areas.
- **A sustainable way of living:** An approach to food and your body that you can maintain through stress, celebrations, illness, ageing, and all the variations of life. You want something that works in the real world, not just under perfect conditions.

Traditional Approaches: Missing Almost Everything You Need

Traditional diets might deliver short-term weight loss, but they fail catastrophically on almost every other need.

They create more food obsession, not less. They destroy your ability to enjoy food by turning it into a moral battleground. They eliminate food as a source of comfort while providing no alternatives. They undermine trust in your judgment by replacing it with external rules. They generate massive shame when they inevitably fail. The skills they teach – restriction, deprivation, and rigid control – don't transfer to other areas of your life in healthy ways. And they're completely unsustainable, which is why you regain the weight plus more.

Now let's examine why every approach you've encountered fails to deliver this complete package.

Weight-Loss Medications: A Partial Solution

Medications like GLP-1 can deliver weight loss and reduce food obsession temporarily, but they don't teach you to enjoy food without guilt, use it for comfort appropriately, or trust your own judgment. When the medication stops working or becomes unavailable, you're left without any of the skills you need. The weight often returns because your underlying relationship with food hasn't healed. You may feel powerful while on the medication, but dependent and powerless when you consider life without it.

Bariatric Surgery: Mechanical Without Psychological

Surgery can provide significant weight loss and force portion control, but it often increases shame and fear around food rather than reducing it. You can't enjoy eating when you're terrified of your body's mechanical limitations.

The surgery doesn't teach emotional regulation skills, so you lose food as a comfort tool without gaining alternatives. Many people struggle with feeling they 'cheated' to lose weight, which undermines rather than builds confidence and personal power.

Intuitive Eating: Right Goal, Wrong Timing

Intuitive eating principles – developing a peaceful relationship with food based around listening to your body's natural hunger and fullness cues – represent where you want to end up: trusting your body, enjoying food, eating without obsession. But for someone with Sensible Sobriety Seeker patterns, it often fails to deliver weight loss, which remains a legitimate need. Without addressing the neurobiological damage caused by years of restriction, simply trying to eat intuitively can feel chaotic and out of control. The shame patterns remain unaddressed, so 'mistakes' can still trigger catastrophic self-loathing. Many people gain weight initially when they start intuitive eating, which reinforces their belief that they can't trust themselves.

Health at Every Size (HAES): Philosophy Without Practical Tools

HAES approaches – that move away from weight as the primary indicator of health – address shame and promote body acceptance, which are crucial needs. But they often dismiss weight loss as a goal entirely, which doesn't meet your legitimate desire to lose weight. Without providing structured alternatives to restriction, many people feel lost and end up either continuing to restrict in secret or eating chaotically. The approach doesn't specifically address the addiction-like patterns that drive Sensible Sobriety Seeking.

Traditional Therapy: Insight Without Neurobiological Tools

Therapy can address underlying trauma and build emotional skills, which are essential. But most therapists don't understand the specific neurobiological patterns of Sensible Sobriety Seeking. Talk therapy alone rarely delivers weight loss or specifically addresses food obsession. Many therapists inadvertently shame patients for wanting weight loss, rather than working with this legitimate goal. Without addressing the addiction-like aspects of the relationship with food, insight alone often isn't enough to create change.

Eating Disorder (ED) Treatment: Close But Not Quite

Eating disorder treatment understands disordered patterns and addresses shame, which is crucial. But traditional ED treatment focuses heavily on mental health and often requires you to abandon weight-loss goals entirely, which doesn't meet your needs. Many programmes are designed for restrictive disorders and don't fully address the binge eating component of Sensible Sobriety Seeking. The abstinence from diet culture, while necessary, often doesn't provide structured alternatives for someone whose internal regulation is severely disrupted.

Support Groups: Community Without Complete Solutions

Groups like Overeaters Anonymous provide community and address the addiction-like aspects of disordered eating, which are important. But they often promote lifelong powerlessness over food rather than building genuine empowerment. The rigid food rules many groups advocate can trigger the same restriction-rebellion cycles. Weight loss isn't typically a focus, so they don't meet your complete needs; and the 'one size fits all' approach doesn't take individual neurobiological differences into account.

Mindful Eating: Good Practice, Missing Pieces

Mindful eating – in which you practise being fully attentive to your food, eating, and hunger and satiety cues – can help rebuild awareness and enjoyment of food, which are important goals. But for someone with severely disrupted hunger and fullness signals, mindfulness alone often doesn't provide enough structure. The approach doesn't specifically address weight-loss goals. Without first addressing the addiction-like patterns, mindful eating can feel overwhelming or trigger anxiety about being 'out of control'.

Exercise Programmes: Physical Without Psychological

Exercise can improve mood, health, and sometimes support weight loss. But for Sensible Sobriety Seekers, exercise often becomes another form of punishment or control rather than enjoyment. These programmes don't address food obsession, shame, or your underlying relationship with food. Exercise alone rarely addresses emotional eating patterns or builds the food-specific skills you need.

The Gap That Nothing Fills

Every approach you've tried succeeds in some areas while failing in others. Traditional diets might provide short-term weight loss but destroy your relationship with food. Therapy might address underlying issues but ignore your legitimate weight concerns. Intuitive eating might restore food enjoyment but doesn't deliver weight loss. Medication might suppress appetite but not build lasting skills.

What's missing is an approach that:

- Recognizes weight loss as a legitimate goal while healing your relationship with food.
- Addresses the neurobiological damage caused by years of restriction-binge cycles, providing enough structure for someone whose internal regulation is disrupted while helping you move towards genuine autonomy.
- Specifically targets the shame that drives Sensible Sobriety Seeker patterns, acknowledging your unique vulnerabilities and working with them rather than against them.
- Treats the addiction-like aspects of your relationship with both restriction and bingeing, building skills that transfer to other life areas, creating genuine empowerment.

HOW DIETS MAKE US FAT

- Works in real-world conditions, not just perfect environments.

You need an approach based on addiction recovery principles, because that's what actually works for people whose relationship with food has been systematically destroyed and rebuilt around dependency and shame. Unlike other approaches that either ignore weight concerns completely or make weight loss the sole focus, this framework will show you how to meet all your needs simultaneously – healing your relationship with food while naturally supporting your body's healthiest weight; building genuine empowerment while addressing neurobiological realities; creating sustainable change while working with your unique brain rather than against it.

The solution isn't to try harder at approaches that only meet some of your needs. It's to finally use a framework designed to meet all of them – because you deserve nothing less than complete recovery.

Chapter 15

A Different Kind of Recovery

You don't need more willpower. You don't need another diet. You don't need to learn to love your body before you can change it. What you need is recovery from addiction – not to food, but to restriction, to bingeing, to the emotional rollercoaster of diet culture, and to using your relationship with food as a way to manage unbearable shame.

But this isn't like traditional addiction recovery where you abstain completely from the substance. You can't stop eating. But you *can* recover.

Why Addiction Recovery Principles Work

Addiction recovery succeeds where other approaches fail because it understands something fundamental: when someone's brain has been rewired by repeated exposure to addictive patterns, you can't simply reason, motivate, or inspire your way out. You need specific strategies designed to work with altered neurobiology, not against it.

Addiction recovery doesn't expect perfection from day one. It builds in support for difficult moments and treats every slip as information rather than failure. It focuses on building genuine capabilities rather than relying on motivation that inevitably fluctuates. Most importantly, addiction recovery understands that shame is the enemy of change. It actively works to reduce shame because it knows that shame creates the exact conditions that make addictive behaviors more likely.

This Isn't Traditional Food Addiction Treatment

When most people hear the term food addiction, they think of someone who can't control themselves around certain foods – usually sugar or processed foods. Traditional food addiction approaches often involve complete abstinence from trigger foods, rigid meal plans, and viewing yourself as permanently powerless over certain substances. But what you're dealing with is more complex than simple food addiction. This means your recovery can't be about avoiding certain foods or following those rigid meal plans. It has to address all the addictive components simultaneously while still allowing you to lose weight and live in the real world where food is everywhere.

These are the three core addictions we're addressing . . .

- **Addiction to Restriction:** You've become dependent on the feeling of control, virtue, and moral superiority that comes from successfully restricting food. This addiction is powerful because restriction temporarily relieves shame while creating a sense of purpose and identity. The problem is that restriction is biologically unsustainable, so the relief is always temporary, requiring increasingly extreme measures to achieve the same psychological reward.
- **Addiction to Bingeing:** After periods of restriction, bingeing provides neurochemical relief through the flood of pleasure chemicals and the psychological relief of stopping the fight against hunger. But bingeing also drives emotional numbing – a way to dissociate from overwhelming feelings of shame, anxiety, or pain. This addiction is particularly challenging because eating is necessary for survival, so you can't simply avoid it entirely.
- **Addiction to the Cycle Itself:** The anticipation of transformation, the early success, the hope and excitement of a fresh start. Even the shame after 'failing' that provides an opportunity for the experience of beginning again.

How This Recovery Is Different

Unlike traditional addiction recovery where you abstain from the substance, your recovery involves learning to have a completely different relationship with food while still eating it every day. This requires specific adaptations:

- **Gradual exposure rather than complete avoidance:** Instead of eliminating trigger foods permanently, you'll learn to gradually reintroduce them while building skills to handle them differently. This is necessary because complete food avoidance is impossible in real life and often reinforces the addiction to restriction.
- **Building tolerance rather than maintaining abstinence:** Your goal isn't to never feel triggered by food, but to build your capacity to be around food without automatically engaging in addictive patterns. This means learning to sit with discomfort, manage cravings, and make conscious choices even when you feel pulled towards familiar patterns.
- **Working with biology rather than against it:** Traditional addiction recovery often involves fighting cravings and urges. But your food cravings are often biologically appropriate responses to restriction. Instead of fighting them, you'll learn to understand what they're telling you and respond appropriately, which often means eating more, not less.
- **Addressing shame as the primary driver:** Most addiction recovery focuses on the behavior itself. But your addictive patterns are driven primarily by shame, which means shame reduction becomes the central therapeutic target. As shame decreases, the need for both restriction and bingeing as coping mechanisms naturally diminishes.

HOW DIETS MAKE US FAT

What Recovery Actually Looks Like

Recovery from Sensible Sobriety Seeking doesn't mean you'll never think about food or your body again. It means food stops being the central organizing principle of your life. You'll still have preferences, goals, and values around eating, but they'll come from a place of self-care rather than self-punishment.

You'll learn to eat regularly without extreme restriction, managing the anxiety that comes with giving up rigid control, and building alternative coping strategies for emotional distress. You'll practise tolerance – sitting with the discomfort of not following familiar patterns while your brain rewires itself.

You'll learn to recognize hunger and fullness signals as they gradually return. You'll practise eating for pleasure without guilt. You'll build a diverse toolkit of emotional regulation strategies. You'll navigate social situations and stressful periods without automatically reverting to addictive patterns.

Eventually, weight management becomes possible because you're no longer fighting your biology. As your relationship with food normalizes, your body's natural weight regulation systems can function. Weight loss, if appropriate for your body, happens as a natural consequence of eating in a way that serves your overall wellbeing rather than as the primary goal that drives disordered behaviors.

The Skills That Transfer

One of the most powerful aspects of this recovery approach is that the skills you develop around food transfer to every other area of your life. Learning to tolerate discomfort without immediately reaching for a coping mechanism improves your capacity to handle work stress, relationship challenges, and life's inevitable difficulties. Building genuine self-compassion changes the way you treat yourself in all areas, not just around food. Developing the ability to make values-based choices rather than fear-based choices transforms your entire approach to decision-making.

Why This Works

This approach succeeds where others have failed because it addresses the complete picture of what's happened to you. It doesn't ignore your desire for weight loss or dismiss it as vanity. It doesn't pretend that willpower alone can overcome neurobiological programming. It doesn't assume that you can simply return to 'normal' eating when normal was systematically destroyed years ago.

Instead, it provides a comprehensive framework for rebuilding your relationship with food from the ground up, while working with your brain's current wiring rather than against it. It treats your struggles as logical responses to systematic programming rather than evidence of personal weakness. And it focuses on building genuine empowerment rather than simply managing symptoms.

What to Expect from This Journey

Recovery is not linear. You'll have days when everything feels easy and natural, and days when you feel pulled back towards familiar patterns. This is normal and expected, not evidence of failure. Each challenging moment is an opportunity to practise your recovery skills and prove to yourself that you can handle difficult situations without reverting to addictive behaviors.

I know you want this fixed immediately. You're wired for intensity and dramatic change – that's part of what made you vulnerable to diet culture in the first place, and it's also part of what will make you successful in recovery. The good news is that you'll start seeing and feeling changes quickly. Within days, you'll notice shifts in your relationship with food. Within weeks, you'll have tangible proof that this approach is different. Within months, you'll have skills that fundamentally change how you navigate food and emotions.

The changes happen faster than you expect because you're finally working with your brain's wiring. Your intensity, your all-or-nothing thinking, your craving for transformation – these aren't character flaws to overcome. They're superpowers to harness. Where diet culture exploited these traits to keep you trapped, recovery channels them to set you free.

But here's what's different: unlike diets that give you quick results followed by inevitable failure, this approach gives you quick relief from food obsession and emotional chaos, followed by increasingly stable progress. You'll feel better fast, and then you'll keep feeling better. The dramatic transformation you've always craved will actually happen – it will just look different than you expected.

Most importantly, recovery is not about becoming a different person. It's about returning to who you always were underneath the programming of diet culture. The person who can trust their body, enjoy food, and make decisions from a place of self-care rather than self-punishment has always been there. Recovery is simply the process of removing the layers of conditioning that have buried your authentic self. So, if you're ready, let's begin . . .

PART 3

THE WAY OUT

Chapter 16

The Beginning of Behavioral Change

What Dieting Actually Asks of You

What you're about to read is not the beginning of another diet. It's the beginning of your journey to freedom from the rules, logic, shame, and confusion that have made change feel impossible.

This section does promise weight loss. But that weight loss is not going to happen because, suddenly, you're going to stick to the plans you've been given your whole life. This isn't about finally staying 'good' forever. It's about real behavioral change – the kind that diet culture pretends to teach but never does. The kind that means you don't have to think about food all day. The expectations diet culture imposes are not just hard; they are the toughest possible behavioral demands.

HOW DIETS MAKE US FAT

If I wanted to design a process that guaranteed failure but still kept you buying, I would take a goal of incredible emotional value (thinness) and make achieving it technically simple but behaviorally brutal. Done.

You are not just trying to change habits. You are trying to:
- Prioritize thinness over pleasure, hunger, convenience, and peace – over and over, every day
- Override your impulses and hunger without relief or visible results later on
- Stay committed to something that hasn't worked
- Remain faithful to a purchased diet plan through exhaustion, confusion, and pain, when every instinct tells you to do whatever you like
- Ignore the part of you that suspects none of this is working (the same part that's kept you alive)
- Sustain extreme effort indefinitely without knowing when relief will come or if it will work
- Withstand streaks of restriction without knowing how long they need to last or if they'll pay off
- Eat rigidly and morally, the opposite of how humans are designed to eat
- Say 'no' to food in a world that celebrates through consumption, making you always the odd one out
- Replace spontaneity, joy, flexibility, comfort, familiarity, and connection, with willpower alone

And then you're told that if you can't do all this, *you* are the problem.

But what if you're not? What if the reason you can't

do what's asked is because your brain and body are doing exactly what they're designed to do? What if the part of you that keeps 'failing' is the part that's keeping you alive?

Scarcity in Disguise

Most people associate scarcity with starvation and poverty. But dieting creates a behavioral and psychological scarcity that functions in exactly the same way. It asks you to live in famine while being surrounded by a feast. You know there's food everywhere – but you're not allowed to have it. Not the kind you want. Not the kind that brings you joy. Not the kind that feels enough. And so even if you're eating, you're still living in famine, but a voluntary famine.

Your body doesn't know the difference. It responds the same way animals have always responded to famine: bingeing, storing, obsessing, prioritizing high-calorie food, preparing for more scarcity. Not because it's broken. Because it's working. But diet culture tells you that your job is to keep choosing famine. This is not sustainable and it's not behavioral change. It's often chronic malnourishment disguised as control.

Why it never stuck

You've probably spent years telling yourself:
- I'm weak
- I sabotage myself
- I can never stick to anything

HOW DIETS MAKE US FAT

In reality, you should be saying:
- I can't keep making thinness the most important thing in the world every time I eat
- I can't keep following boring rules forever when nothing's changing fast enough to justify the misery
- I need food and my choices to feel exciting, not punishing, because joy matters
- I can't keep pretending that moderation works when it only leads to rebellion

If Weight Loss Were Just Behavioral Change

If weight loss wasn't wrapped up in diet culture, it would be treated like every other difficult skill you've ever had to build:
- You'd expect discomfort at first
- You'd know that progress is uneven
- You'd assume you'd make mistakes and learn from them
- You'd get better with practise
- You'd trust that even hard things become easier with time
- You wouldn't moralize your failures
- You wouldn't quit just because it didn't work perfectly the first time

Weight loss made eating personal. Dieting made it moral and humiliating to struggle. It convinced you that failure proved you were weak rather than human.

And here's the kicker: if you can't meet diet culture's standards – if you can't stay hungry forever, avoid every celebration, obey every rule, ignore every craving, sacrifice every joy – that's not a failure. That's actually a great sign that your behavioral system is still functioning.

Resistance Is the Proof You're Still In There

If it feels impossible to stick to the rules of diet culture, that's good. It means your brain still protects you. Your body still wants safety. Your mind still wants joy. Your hunger still matters. Your instincts aren't gone.

From here, you can start building skill and genuine long-lasting behavioral change. It's hard, yes – but it's the kind of hard that does end; because it gets easier; because it builds mastery; and because it's built for you, not for someone else.

This is not about becoming someone who finally follows the rules. This is about unlearning the rules that never made sense and finally getting what you wanted all along. This is not the beginning of another try. This is the beginning of the end of trying. This understanding – that you're facing behavioral challenges made intentionally difficult by diet culture's design – is essential before you begin the actual framework. Because what you're about to learn isn't another set of rules to follow perfectly. It's a complete system for remembering what you've always been capable of.

Chapter 17
The Power Recovery Framework

The Eagle

Before I explain the framework itself, I need you to understand something about your true nature. Let me tell you a story that was shared with me when working in addiction treatment, as a tool for helping service users to remember their capacity.

Once upon a time, a man found an eagle's egg and placed it under a brooding hen. The eaglet hatched among the chickens and grew up believing he was one of them. He clucked and cackled, scratched the earth for worms, flapped his wings just enough to lift a few feet off the ground, and that became his truth.

One day the eagle looked up and saw a magnificent bird in the sky: effortless, powerful, gliding in full command of the wind. Captivated, he asked: 'Who's that?'

'That's the eagle,' replied one of the chickens. 'That's the king of the birds. He belongs to the sky. But we're chickens. We belong here.'

And so the eagle stayed on the ground, never questioning it again, because that's what he had been taught. By then, he couldn't imagine himself to be anything other.

You are that eagle. You've spent your entire life in the chicken pen of diet culture, learning to see yourself as fundamentally flawed, broken, lacking in willpower. You've been taught that your natural instincts around food can't be trusted, that your body is the enemy, that you need external rules and restrictions to keep yourself in line. You've been conditioned to believe that losing weight requires punishment, deprivation, and constant vigilance against your own supposedly weak character.

But here's what nobody told you: you were never a chicken. You were always an eagle who simply forgot how to fly.

The Glimpses of Flight You've Already Had

You've known you can fly for a while. You've accidentally managed to flap your wings enough times to get a glimpse of the sky: those moments when eating felt natural, when you stopped when you were satisfied, when food was just fuel and pleasure rather than a source of shame and struggle. You saw how different life looked from up there compared to the pen.

But then, as soon as the wind changed or you didn't know how to navigate the currents, you forgot you were that eagle and panicked about how high up you were. You didn't know how to survive and couldn't imagine a time when it would get easier. You never got to really enjoy it, but you briefly realized that it was technically possible, you caught a glimpse of freedom, and you saw that eagle life was far better than chicken life.

So you kept falling to the ground, chasing that first flight. Every diet, every 'fresh start', every Monday morning promise to be different this time have all been attempts to get back to that sky you glimpsed. But every time you got there and managed to stay a little longer, everything reminded you that the crash back to the pen was imminent. The real betrayal is that no one told you the truth: you can fly, but no one taught you how to stay in the sky because your wings never developed.

Flight School

This framework is your flight school. It's not another set of rules to follow perfectly, not another diet disguised as wisdom, but a complete system for remembering what you've always been capable of.

I'm going to teach you not just how to get to the sky, but how to *live* there; how to navigate storms, how to find food when you need it, how to rest when you're tired, and how to soar when the conditions are right.

The Inner Conflict

This is the war inside you: your reflective, rational brain knows diets don't work, but your automatic, emotional brain is still responding to old fears, habits, and diet-culture programming. Understanding why these two parts of your brain can be at odds is key to healing your relationship with food. This isn't about willpower or motivation – it's about how your brain naturally operates when it encounters the modern food environment.

Your Reflective Brain (Planning System)

This is the part of your brain that thinks, plans, and evaluates long-term consequences. It can read, analyze, and understand patterns. It sees clearly that dieting often leads to restriction, bingeing, and frustration. It recognizes that sustainable change happens gradually and that self-compassion is more effective than self-criticism.

When you're calm and well-resourced, this system can guide your decisions, helping you make balanced choices and honour your body's needs.

Your Automatic Brain (Acting System)

This is the part of your brain that responds quickly to environmental cues and immediate emotional signals. It operates from habit, emotion, and survival instincts, not logic. It remembers what worked – or didn't – in the past and often overrides the reflective brain in moments of stress, fatigue, or strong cravings.

Your automatic brain isn't 'bad' or lazy – it's doing what it evolved to do: prioritizing safety, reward, and survival in a world that historically had far fewer cues and temptations than today. The challenge is that this system reacts to patterns that no longer serve you, but it cannot yet know that.

Why Some Approaches Fail

Most programmes try to convince your acting system with logic or information. This is like trying to calm a frightened child by explaining statistics – it ignores what the emotional, automatic brain actually responds to: repeated experience and evidence that it can relax its protective behaviors.

The Strategy

We don't convince this part of the brain with facts – we show it through repeated, safe experiences that food is not a threat:
- Food is abundant and available whenever you need it
- You can stop when you're satisfied
- You can cope with emotions without relying on food
- All foods are safe, even the ones you currently struggle with
- You can maintain a weight that feels healthy without constant restriction
- You can take care of yourself with kindness, not cruelty

Understanding Food Chatter and Food Noise

Food chatter is the automatic brain signalling that it perceives risk. It's not a moral failing – it's information about what it's worried about. By showing it safe, successful experiences, you 'update' this system to understand that restriction, deprivation, and panic aren't necessary anymore.

The goal isn't to silence the automatic brain – it's to make its responses predictable, impersonal, and neutral. The more you practise safe, consistent behavior, the less reactive it becomes, turning once-anxious signals into ordinary noise.

Food Noise: Your Brain's Alert System

Before I explain the framework components, you need to understand what food noise actually is, because this understanding completely changes the way you relate to it.

Food noise is evidence that you've gone back into your automatic brain. It's an alert that something has happened. Forgetting that you can choose what you want, and that food isn't more powerful than you are, is actually a call to action that we should be grateful for.

When food noise increases, that automatic part is worried about you. It worries you'll suffer, doesn't know what's coming next, and only has the past as reference. It's operating from the exact emotional place where hunger was first imposed without understanding why – knowing only that something was wrong and food became bad, something to be taken away.

This automatic part has watched you try to starve repeatedly. It's seen you hurt, disappointed, ill, confused, jittery, every time your dieting went too far. It's witnessed your struggles, and it's scared you'll eventually succeed at starving long enough to harm yourself.

Food noise – 'you shouldn't eat this,' 'you can't be trusted,' 'this won't work' – isn't just being mean. Your automatic brain doesn't want you to succeed at starvation. It tells you what it thinks will prevent restriction success.

The Four Conditions for Food Noise Quiet

Through working with hundreds of people and examining what actually creates lasting weight management, I've identified four conditions that must exist simultaneously for food noise to quiet:

- Not being physically hungry at the wrong times
- Not emotionally craving
- Following a plan that delivers results while removing decision-making burden
- Learning to handle foods that currently feel chaotic

If you've experienced fast results from medications or appetite suppression, you recognize this pattern: they work by artificially creating these conditions. They remove physical hunger, reduce emotional craving, remove decision-making burden (fewer food decisions needed), and quiet challenging food noise (less frequent encounters with shame-activating foods).

But you haven't learned the skills needed to create these conditions yourself, which is why weight often returns rapidly when external suppression ends.

The Ten-Step Framework Structure

The Power Recovery Framework systematically creates these four conditions through ten interconnected steps:

- Step 1: Power Assessment – Understanding your daily capacity for making kind decisions and choosing appropriate approaches based on your actual bandwidth
- Step 2: Creating Your Baseline – Building your maintenance-first eating approach, designed from the end goal backwards
- Step 3: The Bridge Days – Your crisis management system that prevents temporary struggles from becoming permanent setbacks
- Step 4: Building Your Flight Record – Your detailed curriculum for unlearning chaos-creating behaviors and learning empowering ones
- Step 5: Reclaiming Your Hands – Maintaining agency and choice even during difficult moments, preventing the victim mentality that keeps you stuck
- Step 6: Reclaiming Forbidden Territory – Strategic approaches to challenging and trigger foods, deciding when to include versus exclude
- Step 7: Changing Your Internal Script – Transforming your critical internal voice into a supportive guide that expects difficulty as part of learning
- Step 8: Emotional Regulation Without Food – Developing skills to process difficult emotions without using food as your primary coping mechanism
- Step 9: Real-Life Application – Navigating social situations, travel, and complex scenarios that don't fit neatly into other categories

- Step 10: Long-Term Maintenance and Your Comprehensive Toolkit – Sustaining your progress and continuing to build evidence of capability across all life circumstances

These aren't sequential steps you complete and abandon. They're ongoing tools used simultaneously, scaling based on your power and circumstances, continuously building evidence that you can trust yourself around food regardless of what's happening in your life.

We Need to Be Succeeding

Remember: we need to feel successful long enough to get good at something. Then we can ride on being good at it.

Your body does the opposite of sabotaging when it's hungry or craving. Your mind does the opposite of sabotaging because food noise was learned to keep you safe. You only call it sabotage because not eating is applauded in your society.

All you ever need to do is make the next best choice. All habit change is one choice after another, in a row, until it's easier. Choices come from noise – internal noise, food noise, confusion, legacy thinking ('it's a fluke'), weight-loss thoughts, self-doubt, memories of failure, low self-belief, making food worse because you've made weight worse, all-or-nothing commands.

This framework gives you constant opportunities to succeed, build capability evidence, and make the next best choice easier every time.

Chapter 18

Step 1 – Power Assessment

Understanding Your Daily Capacity

The most important concept in this entire framework is this: not every day is the same, and expecting consistent performance from yourself – regardless of your actual capacity – is setting yourself up for failure.

Step 1 teaches you how to assess your daily power and choose an appropriate approach based on your real capacity rather than wishful thinking. This prevents the biggest trap that sabotages sustainable change: trying to maintain the same standards regardless of your fluctuating daily levels of default power.

What You Must Accept About This Process

Before we dive into the daily power assessment, you need to accept some fundamental truths that will change how you approach every food decision.

Long-term freedom is only possible when you take power out of the food noise learned from diet culture. Not only to be nicer to yourself, but because the food choices, states, and beliefs created by wrapping eating up in weight loss – and the internal pushback you get as a result – exhausts you, depletes you, and makes you look for comfort in food or control. Both end up in weight gain, one way or another, and they're also responsible for your weight-gaining and powerless eating behaviors.

The only thing you can't do is keep up plans because of the way you've come to view food choices and moralize them and behave around food as a result of it being wrapped up in weight loss.

What You Actually Need to Change

This is it. This is how you actually lose weight and keep it off.

Not through another diet. Not through more restriction. Not through finding the 'right' plan or the 'perfect' foods or the latest supplement. You lose weight and keep it off by learning to eliminate food noise.

Food noise – that relentless mental chatter about what to eat, when you last ate, what you shouldn't eat, and whether you've 'blown it' – isn't just annoying background static. It's the primary driver of weight gain and the reason that every diet you've tried has failed.

Here's why: Food noise creates the chaos that leads to impulsive eating. Impulsive eating creates shame and guilt. Shame and guilt drive you to eat more to numb those feelings. Eating based on shame can drive rapid weight gain. Weight gain creates more food noise ('I'm so fat,' 'I need to lose weight,' 'I can't eat that'). More food noise creates more chaos, and the cycle continues, getting worse each time.

Every failed diet, every 'I'll start Monday,' every moment you've felt powerless around food – it all goes back to food noise.

The Ultimate Goal: Quiet = Power

When your head is completely quiet around food, you have your full power available. You're not wasting mental energy on internal food warfare. You're not spending your day negotiating with yourself about what to eat, beating yourself up about what you've already eaten, or planning how to 'make up' for choices you regret.

Maximum quiet equals maximum power. Maximum power equals remembering you can do whatever you choose to with your hands, remembering that habit change is hard, making decisions you'd like to have made easy already when it's hardest to do so, chasing mastery and ease, feeling smart, wise and mature, not making choices you wouldn't recommend to someone you love, not feeling powerless and hurried and 'possessed'.

Maximum quiet comes when you focus on building power through evidence – not only that it gets easier if you keep doing it, but also evidence that the internal message 'I can't do it' isn't compelling for long when you realize that you *have* been doing it. That's the thing about self-talk: it's really tough to make it kind, but not as tough as turning it fair and factual.

What to Expect

Before we dive into power assessment, I need to prepare you for what this journey actually looks like. Because if you're expecting your food noise to simply fade away quietly and stay gone, you're going to think you're failing when you're actually succeeding.

Food noise doesn't disappear in a straight line. It gets louder, then quieter, then louder again in different areas until eventually it's quiet everywhere. When you start addressing physical hunger – eating regularly, planning ahead, managing your blood-sugar level – the food noise around 'I'm starving, I need something now' will get quieter. But the emotional craving noise might get louder because you're no longer using hunger-driven chaos to avoid difficult feelings.

As you start working on emotional cravings – identifying triggers, building new coping strategies – the noise around using food for comfort and control will start to quiet down. But the decision-making noise might amplify because you're suddenly faced with having to actually choose what to eat instead of defaulting to chaos or restriction.

When you build a sustainable-eating plan – one that delivers results through habit-building rather than body metrics – the noise around 'am I doing this right' and 'is this working' will diminish. But the noise around trigger foods might become deafening because you're no longer avoiding them through complete restriction or surrendering to them through binges.

Finally addressing trigger foods – learning to either include them skilfully or exclude them strategically without shame – will make that specific noise quiet down. But then you'll notice noise in areas you didn't even realize were noisy, like eating in social situations or making choices when your routine is disrupted.

Food Noise That Keeps You Trapped

Before we dive into power assessment, you need to understand exactly what food noise sounds like and why each type creates the chaos that leads to weight gain . . .

1. Physical Hunger Noise

This is the noise that comes from your body's actual need for fuel, but it's been distorted by years of chaotic eating patterns. It sounds like:

- 'I'm starving, I need something NOW'
- 'I can't think straight, where's the nearest food'
- 'I'm so hungry I could eat anything'
- 'I waited too long, now I'm going to make terrible choices'

2. Emotional Craving Noise

This is the noise that comes from trying to use food to manage feelings you don't know how to handle otherwise. It sounds like:

- 'I've had such a stressful day, I deserve this'
- 'I'm so bored, food will make me feel better'
- 'I can't cope with this feeling, I need chocolate'
- 'Everyone else is having fun with food, why can't I?'

3. Decision-Making Noise

This is the noise that comes from constantly having to choose what to eat while carrying the psychological baggage of thousands of previous food decisions that led to shame and weight gain. It sounds like:
- 'What should I have for lunch?'
- 'Is this healthy enough?'
- 'Am I making a good choice?'
- 'Should I eat now or wait?'
- 'What if I regret this later?'

4. Shame-Spiral Noise

This is the noise that comes from foods that carry too much psychological baggage from years of diet failures and 'good food/bad food' thinking. It sounds like:
- 'I shouldn't eat this'
- 'This is going to make me gain weight'
- 'I'm being bad'
- 'I've blown it now'
- 'One bite and I'll eat the whole thing'

Understanding How Food Noise Actually Works

For failed dieters who feel like failures, who carry shame and guilt, and eat on that shame and guilt in an endless spiral that makes everything worse, the insight about appetite suppressants isn't that they make you less hungry.

It's that they quiet the shame cycle that drives chronic weight gain.

Here's what's actually happening: when you're not physically hungry, you're not eating impulsively. When you're not eating impulsively, you're not eating 'badly'. When you're not eating 'badly', you're not feeling guilty. When you're not feeling guilty, you're not eating on that guilt. When you're not eating on guilt, you're not gaining weight from shame-driven binges. When you're not gaining weight, you're not feeling more ashamed. The cycle breaks.

This section will teach you how to create these same conditions without depending on external intervention.

The Universal Challenge

Before we move into power assessment, there's something crucial you need to understand: much of the food noise you experience isn't because you're broken or have a 'food addiction' or lack willpower. It's because you're a human being trying to eat healthily in a world designed to make that difficult.

When I refer to people who don't have a complicated relationship with food, I'm talking about people who have never been on repeated diets, who don't moralize their food choices, who eat when hungry and stop when satisfied without drama, and who don't associate their eating with their self-worth. Even these people experience food noise.

They get fed up with meal planning. They feel guilty when they spend money on unhealthy food choices. They get frustrated when they haven't thought ahead and they've ended up making choices they regret. The difference is in how they interpret this difficulty.

When someone without a complicated relationship with food finds meal planning boring, they think, 'Ugh, meal planning is boring, but I need to do it anyway.' When you find meal planning boring, you think, 'This is so hard, I'm failing again, maybe I'm just not cut out for this, I should give up.' This interpretation difference happens because you've spent years associating any difficulty around food and health with diet failure, restriction, and rebellion.

Learning to separate 'this is hard because it's genuinely hard for everyone' from 'this is hard because I'm fundamentally flawed' is essential for sustainable change.

Your Daily Power Assessment

Every morning, before you even think about food, you're going to ask yourself one simple question: 'How equipped am I to make kind food and life decisions today?'

This question is specifically designed to help you tune into your actual capacity rather than what you think you should be capable of. It's not asking whether you want to make good choices – it's asking whether you have the resources to make kind choices consistently throughout the day.

Notice that the question asks about 'kind' decisions rather than 'perfect' decisions. This is deliberate. Perfect decisions require maximum bandwidth because they involve overriding desires, ignoring cravings, and maintaining rigid control.

Kind decisions are about treating yourself with compassion while still supporting your goals.

Start by rating yourself on a scale of 1–10, but this isn't about judgment; it's about information gathering. A low score isn't a failure; it's valuable data that helps you make appropriate plans for the day.

The Factors That Determine Your Power

Physical factors include your sleep quality, nutrition, hormonal fluctuations, wellness, exercise, and basic physical comfort. When your body is well-rested, well-fed, and feeling good, you have more resources available for handling challenges.

Emotional factors include your stress levels, relationships, mood, recent experiences, what you need emotionally today. When you're feeling calm, supported, and emotionally stable, you can handle much more than when you're anxious, lonely, overwhelmed, or dealing with difficult emotions.

Mental factors include your workload, decision fatigue, how much mental focus you need today, and cognitive demands. When your mental resources aren't overtaxed, you have capacity for additional challenges.

Environmental factors include your surroundings, social pressures, obligations, disruptions to your routine, and external stressors. When your environment is supportive and predictable, you can take more risks.

All these factors interact with each other. Poor sleep affects your emotional regulation, which affects your decision-making, which affects your ability to handle stress, which affects your relationships, which affects your mood, which affects your sleep.

Your Three-Track System

Based on your daily power assessment, you'll follow one of three tracks . . .

Track 1: Bridge Days (Power Level 1–4)

Your worst-day plan, designed for maximum self-care and minimum chaos-inducing foods. Nothing that typically creates problems for you, maximum comfort, acting like someone who hasn't developed a complicated relationship with food. These days protect your Baseline by preventing you from associating it with periods when you were struggling.

Track 2: Baseline Days (Power Level 5–10)

Your maintenance-first eating plan, designed for keeping weight off, not getting there. This is how you eat when you're not trying to lose weight as quickly as possible and you're not rebelling against impossible rules. This is where you do the majority of your evidence collection and prove to yourself that you can make food choices from a calm place.

Track 3: Challenge Days (Power Level 8–10+ and Your Baseline Feels Solid)

Opportunities to test yourself with more challenging situations when you feel strong and your Baseline is already working consistently. These are the days when you expand your comfort zone and build evidence that you can handle increasingly complex food situations. But they should only happen when *both* conditions are met: high power *and* established Baseline confidence. Don't attempt Challenge Days in your first weeks of building your Baseline, even if your power feels high.

Your Morning Power Protocol

Every morning, this is what you do:
- Assess power: Rate yourself 1–10 on your capacity for kind decisions
- Choose your track: Baseline (5–10) or Bridge Days (1–4)
- Check your flight record: What 1–3 things will you focus on today?
- Set your intention: How will you act like someone who trusts themselves around food today?

This routine removes the guesswork and decision fatigue that often lead to poor choices. Instead of waking up wondering what approach to take, you have a clear framework based on your actual capacity.

Important Notes About Power Assessment

Sometimes it will feel as though your power is high because you're losing weight, and you may have underestimated the degree to which that fact in itself is what's making you think your power is high.

The way to know whether your power is high for a reason that will backfire on you (because you've attached food and weight again), or if your power is legitimately high, is to think about your body and where that's at, rather than simply where the food chatter is at. When you say you have more energy, do you mean in spirits for the day or genuine sustained energy? How frequently are you hungry? How likely would you be to keep this up on your worst day?

This distinction is crucial because artificial power – the kind that comes from seeing a good number on the scale or fitting into smaller clothes – is fragile and disappears the moment your weight fluctuates upwards or you have a challenging food day. Real power comes from genuine physical and emotional resources and is much more stable.

Design for Your Worst Day

Think about the last time you completely abandoned all your healthy habits. What was happening in your life? What combination of factors came together to make everything feel impossible?

Most likely, it was a combination of several factors. Your worst days rarely happen because of just one thing – they happen when multiple stressors compound and overwhelm your usual coping capacity.

Your current diet culture default
- **You have a scarcity mindset that drives overeating:** You eat large quantities when 'allowed' foods are available because you expect restriction to return.

HOW DIETS MAKE US FAT

You need tools to prove food abundance is permanent, templates for 'maintenance eating' that remove the feast-or-famine cycle, and cues to recognize scarcity thinking.

- **You can't trust your own hunger and fullness signals**: You either can't feel hunger/fullness or you don't trust these signals because dieting taught you to override them. You need tools to rebuild signal recognition without perfectionism pressure, permission to eat when hungry even if it's 'not time' according to diet rules, and you need to understand that signal rebuilding takes time.
- **You think in all-or-nothing patterns**: You believe one imperfect choice ruins everything, leading to day-long or extended binges. You need individual habit tracking that separates different behaviors, scripts for moments of 'blown it' thinking, and evidence that successful people make imperfect choices and continue normally.
- **You associate food with moral value and shame**: You feel guilty about enjoying food, leading to emotional eating to cope with food-related shame. You need tools to remove moral language around food choices, permission scripts to enjoy food without guilt, and you need to understand that guilt about eating literally drives more eating.
- **You depend on external rules instead of internal wisdom**: You panic when there's no diet plan to follow, leading to chaotic eating until the next restriction. You need a framework for creating

personal sustainable eating patterns, tools to develop internal food wisdom rather than rule-following, and confidence-building through small autonomous food decisions.

- **You live in restriction-rebellion cycles**: You automatically rebel against any structure, even health-supportive structure, because it feels like dieting. You need a clear distinction between health-supportive structure and restrictive dieting, an approach that removes the deprivation mindset, and tools to recognize when rebellion serves you versus when it harms you.
- **You have hyper-vigilant food thoughts (food noise)**: You can't stop thinking about food, what you should/shouldn't eat, planning your next meal or restriction. You need to understand that food noise is protective, not broken thinking, tools to make food thoughts impersonal rather than emotionally charged, and evidence collection that proves you can handle food situations calmly.

Accepting Mastery

You need to accept that your food choices, once separated from each other and treated like any other skill, will get easier – like anything else – once you have gathered evidence.

The evidence gathering is to calm your body, come out unscathed, and build proof that's harder to push back against. But it's also not actually required. If you accept that your changes will eventually come down to one choice in a row, no matter how many choices you need to unlearn/learn/practise, and you accept that each of those choices is doable, and that in a row they will become automatic; if you can remind yourself every single time that you believe in the plan and the formula, then this problem can be over *today*.

In the end this is all about proving to yourself what you already know and what is evident when anyone looks at you.

What You Must Accept About Trust and Planning

Accept that it will be hard and that you have to trust every aspect of your plan and believe it will work. Because once the actual things you have to do, and eat, are there, you need to just believe the version of you that has your most meaningful goals in mind wrote the plan. You can expect a lot of mental pushback saying it won't work, it's not good enough. Nevertheless, you *have* to trust your plan.

I will help you make a plan that gives you the most quiet and the path of least resistance through this whole process, but you need to accept that there will still be triggers throughout, since being full and being hungry can be triggers, as can success and failure at changing health habits. These can all trigger us to do the diet culture things that got us here in the first place.

Accept that if you had never been on a diet you wouldn't have the unwanted behaviors you have around food, the same ones holding you back from making the calm, wise, sensible choices you'd recommend to your child when you're not bingeing or restricting on a perfect plan.

Why This System Builds Unshakeable Self-Trust

You're not just proving you can eat well when everything is perfect – you're proving you can make caring choices when life is difficult, when you're stressed, when things don't go according to plan. This evidence then becomes the foundation of unshakeable self-trust around food. Instead of fearing difficult days because they've historically led to complete chaos, you start to feel confident that you have the tools to handle whatever comes up.

Chapter 19

Step 2 – Creating Your Baseline

Working Backwards

Now that you understand how to assess your daily power and choose an appropriate approach, we need to build your Baseline – the eating plan you'll use most of the time when your power is on point.

If you woke up tomorrow and you were already at your goal weight, what habits, choices, characteristics would you need to be doing, making, demonstrating automatically, in order to stay at that weight easily and without giving it any thought? These are the things that you need to learn and unlearn.

Your Baseline is essentially the way you're going to eat in order to keep off lost weight. It's predictable eating that starts at the end goal and maintenance but addresses challenging foods strategically once your foundation is solid. This approach is fundamentally different because we're not designing this to get you to your goal – we're designing it to keep you there. This distinction changes everything about how we approach food choices, portion sizes, meal timing, and food variety.

Understanding Your Safe Harbour: Your Maintenance-First Eating Plan

Your Baseline is how you eat – what you eat, and when you intend to eat. It's the most important part to separate, and sticking to your Baseline is one of the things to learn in itself, as is staying on track when you haven't been perfect.

This is where you should be most of the time. The only hard thing about it should be the internal pushback about not thinking this plan will work, wanting to ramp it up, and so on, and the challenge of literally planning and cooking and organizing and thinking about meal planning and prep. Other than that, it should be the most varied, thought-out comprehensive collection of foods, including meals, snacks, options from shops/cafes near where you work, and options when you want something sweet.

Your Baseline must feel so sustainable and appealing that you actually look forward to returning to it after periods of going off track. It's not a punishment you have to endure – it's a home base that feels good to come back to.

Why Your Baseline Isn't a Diet

Your Baseline is designed for maintenance, not weight loss. This distinction is crucial because your relationship with your

Baseline determines whether it will work in the long term or become just another diet that you eventually rebel against. These are some of the other differences . . .

- A diet says: 'Follow these rules perfectly to lose weight fast, and if you deviate, you've failed.' A Baseline says: 'These guidelines support your wellbeing, and you can always return to them when you're ready.'
- A diet is temporary: You go on it when you want to lose weight and off it when you reach your goal or give up. A Baseline is permanent: It's how you prefer to live, not a means to an end.
- A diet restricts: It systematically removes foods, food groups, or eating occasions to create a calorific deficit. A Baseline guides: It provides structure while allowing flexibility for real life.
- A diet moralizes: You're good when you follow it perfectly and bad when you don't. A Baseline supports: It's there to serve you, not judge you.
- A diet creates scarcity: It's built on the premise that you can't be trusted around food and need external control. A Baseline creates abundance: It's built on the premise that you can learn to trust yourself and make choices that serve you.
- A diet has an end date: Either when you reach your goal or when you can't stand it anymore. A Baseline evolves: It grows and changes with your life circumstances while maintaining its core principles.

SHAHROO IZADI

The Reality of Food Planning

You have to eat. If you're currently managing to barely eat, then I am sorry to have to break this to you but at some point you will have to make food choices again. Also, eating in a predictable way is a boring and annoying chore for everyone.

I have worked with people in all situations – from those who have to choose what restaurants to go to practically every night to people who work in jobs where hospitality is a reality for breakfast, lunch, and dinner, to people with six children who make everything from scratch, to countless busy professionals who are just so tired of having to think about groceries, what to cook, who eats what, and the dreaded question 'What shall we have for dinner?'

Often when we've been struggling with our weight, we forget that other people find food annoying too. They may not be as bothered as we are about being without it, it may not show up on their bodies in the same way, but it's annoying for anyone to organize what they're going to eat and to have to think about it regularly. Once again you'll just have to accept the reality that this is going to make you feel like you're on a plan – but you're only on a plan because pretty much every human being needs to be on some kind of plan. No one can wing every decision they make about food.

The task here is to make up how you're going to eat. This is the point where we pretend that your trajectory wasn't disrupted in the first place, you were somehow born as an adult, and it's time to decide how and what you're going to eat.

This isn't a manifestation exercise. It is genuinely the only place to start if you don't have a predictable way of eating. Not just as someone with a history of dieting, but as a human being. I know people who haven't had issues with their weight but the boring admin of deciding what to eat and getting organized about it means that, even in the pursuit of being generally healthier, they cannot find a predictable way of eating that they are happy with.

I assure you, my fellow diet culture survivor, this is not a 'you' thing; this is a thing.

What Sort of Eater Do You Wish You Already Were?

We're going to work backwards and help you do this with an exercise that starts with broad strokes. I want you to read these cues and write down your answers . . .

- If someone was describing how I eat most of the time, someone who saw me every day when I wake up in the morning, what I do at lunchtime, for snacks, on holiday, at Christmas, when I order a takeaway, and so on, how would I like them to describe me generally?
- Consider what food identity feels authentic to who you are when you're not trying to lose weight as quickly as possible. What does it look like to eat in a way that feels like you rather than as if you're following someone else's rules?

This question gets at your food identity beyond weight loss. When the pressure to be 'good' is removed and you're in a social situation where you want to be seen as normal and enjoyable to be around, what foods feel authentic to who you are? This helps you think beyond 'diet foods' to foods that you actually want to eat, that feel representative of your personality and preferences.

Think about the events and circumstances where you'd like to see yourself eating delicious foods, delicious foods that you like the idea of keeping in your life provided you feel empowered around them. What would those delicious foods be? What are the foods that you refuse to say goodbye to forever? If you knew there was a way to work with them in a way that was calm and didn't make you spiral or feel guilty?

Because remember, the reason you feel guilty is because you don't want to gain weight from what you've just done; and the reason you gain weight from what you've just done is because you feel guilty; and when you feel guilty, you eat more. This is very important.

This question addresses the foods that you've been trying to eliminate through restriction but that keep pulling you back into chaos. Instead of fighting against these foods forever, we're going to acknowledge that they're part of your authentic food identity and figure out how to include them in a way that doesn't create problems.

- Now I want you to describe the other habits you imagine yourself engaging in when it comes to food specifically, like preparing it, cooking it, being interested in it, the sorts of places you shop, the time you take to cook food, the way you host dinners, the way that the people who love you would describe how you shop for food, your behavior around food, whether you sit at the table, whether you eat while you cook.

Do you want to be someone who enjoys cooking as a creative outlet, or someone who keeps it simple and efficient? Do you want to be someone who sits down for proper meals, or someone who's more casual about eating occasions? Do you want to be someone who loves trying new restaurants, or someone who prefers familiar options?

None of these preferences are right or wrong – they're just different ways of relating to food that should align with your authentic personality and lifestyle. And of course, there is the faintest of silver linings that comes with having tried out a lot of diets – awareness of options.

Making Food Choices Predictable

I want you to think about what you would like to be predictable. I want you to write it out in the same spirit as you thought about your Baseline identity. Because these habits may seem simple, but the habit of keeping them up is hard. All you need is a disruption in momentum for a legitimate reason and the decision to make that meal from scratch, instead of getting a takeaway, becomes very trivial.

But in this moment, there's an important point to make. I want it to seem trivial if we're talking about weight loss.

If you want a delicious takeaway and you've had a stressful day, or for whatever reason you don't want to cook like you said you would, I don't want you to beat yourself up. I want you to have that takeaway, be calm and enjoy it.

But . . . I don't want the fact that you have all these associations with weight loss and failure to hold you back from building healthier habits with food now and for the rest of your life. And that requires making these choices – the ones you would make if weight loss wasn't a consideration. It means choosing to build habits for your health regardless of how you look. And that is something that many of us may have forgotten how to do.

The Importance of Food Planning

I cannot tell you how many clients have told me that batch cooking makes them feel that they have betrayed a rebellious cool fun version of themselves. Then they have come back later and told me that it was absolutely essential.

That one hour spent cooking, and half an hour spent grocery shopping, meant that during their adjustment period, when the all-or-nothing thinking threatened to throw them off track, they were able to remember that they had something in the freezer. Something delicious that they were looking forward to. And then, after they ate, they thought, 'Thank goodness I didn't reach for chocolate and some takeaway. That was lovely and delicious and, more importantly than feeling I've been healthy food wise, I feel I've taken care of myself and backed myself and prepared for myself and it's worked out.' Then of course they have to deal with the backlash of thinking that it was a fluke. Which of course should be one of the main types of pushback that you expect.

The Linking Problem

There is an important reason why we chase results by chasing mastery and breaking down the habits we need to master in order to keep off lost weight. This is because, as we start to build more habits and make more choices, we end up with more new plans and challenges on the go. This means there are also more opportunities for us to feel that we have failed and, as is the case with chronic dieters, feeling we have failed in one domain often makes us feel that we have failed in all domains and act accordingly. That is one of the fundamental things you will need to unlearn.

When weight loss and food choices are inextricably linked, we end up thinking that the choices we make at breakfast dictate the choices we have to make at dinner because we've already been 'bad'. We become convinced that Monday mornings are the only time we can start eating healthy; we stop drinking water because it was part of a restrictive food plan that we've now 'failed at'; we cancel social plans we made, despite wanting to liven up our social lives, because we made them as part of a larger plan to keep us motivated to stay on our diet because having to dress up would give us deadlines.

Linking every food choice is a recipe for disaster if you

don't want to gain weight quickly. Think about it, if we need to make 50 or so food choices per time period at least, if we manage to make 23 and then the 24th one isn't perfect, then the rest of them are all choices that actively cause us to feel powerless, gain weight and eat something 'one last time'.

And the shame of this extends to the fact that if you have been drinking water as part of a restrictive food plan and legitimately building a habit of drinking lots more water every day and feeling good about it, and then you 'fall off' that food plan at a service station and all of a sudden find yourself abandoning your water bottle, you might have been close to that water bottle being a main feature for the rest of your life. But you don't know that because the different behaviors were all being built under the umbrella of losing weight.

When we chase results not by the number on the scales or how we look but by repeating and making easier the choices and habits and practices that enable us to be truly happy with the way we look and what we weigh, we have to separate all the new habits we are building. We are able to go to bed thinking that the challenge of not comfort-eating after work hasn't seen a consistent streak for a while but the challenge of not eating mindlessly in your car and the challenge of making three healthy meals that you enjoy, or the challenge of not throwing in the towel after you made a choice that made you feel guilty, are very much in play. And so you can watch yourself getting better at all these different things and see the long-term process more clearly.

Self-Belief Through Separated Habits

And so now I want you to make a list of all the habits that just have to do with health and generally taking care of yourself, and things that you wish you already found easy to do but you tend to only do if you're losing weight – things like making fresh juice, food planning, batch cooking to make things easier, drinking enough water, exercising, taking supplements, meditating, waking up early, and so on. And I want you to write them down and order them, giving each one a number in terms of how difficult it will be to build this habit. You may find that when you look at them, none of them are difficult to build. What's difficult to build is the habit of feeling it's worth taking care of yourself and building healthy habits when they're not directly connected to a weight-loss goal.

While you build habits, you're building self-belief in the most important part of this, which is the fact that you have the power to practise anything in a row until it becomes easier for you; and that is the only way to learn. But you have a process that factors in difficulty and discomfort and adjustment that you have anticipated and repeated. You have also anticipated the internal and external backlash while you adjust and decided to treat it like any other habit change.

And as is so often the case when our self-esteem and self-worth are attached to short-lived attempts and extreme measures, you will find that when you've built the habit of giving yourself signals that your body matters throughout the day (habits you would have chosen to build just because you want to be a healthy human being), that when you *do* eat unhealthy foods in the future, and even if you *do* have those old feelings of initial guilt, you will be insulated by messages and actions that you have come to normalize. You will be automatically doing certain things for yourself, like reaching for a bottle of water. And all those associations will start to become helpful as the water reminds you that you are no longer necessarily on a mission to lose weight but that you are someone who definitely deserves to be cared for.

Your Baseline Design

As you work through designing your Baseline, you'll need to be specific about different aspects of your eating life. This isn't about creating rigid rules but about establishing preferences and patterns that feel sustainable and appealing.

Think about your Baseline as having multiple components that work together . . .

- **Daily rhythm**: What feels natural for your eating timing, based on your lifestyle, work schedule, and preferences? Some people prefer three meals, others prefer smaller frequent meals, others prefer two larger meals. What feels sustainable for you?
- **Food preferences**: What types of foods genuinely appeal to you and make you feel good physically and emotionally? What cooking methods do you enjoy or find manageable? What do you look forward to that feels safe when it comes to food?

- **Preparation**: How much time and energy do you realistically want to spend on food preparation? What level of planning ahead works for your lifestyle? What shortcuts or conveniences can you build in?
- **Evolution**: How will your Baseline adapt as your life circumstances change? What aspects are non-negotiable versus what can be modified?

Remember: Your Baseline should feel like freedom after the initial adjustment to planning. It should not feel like restriction. It should be a place you genuinely want to return to, your 'way of eating', not something you have to force yourself to maintain. If any aspect feels genuinely unsustainable, even once you've got used to it, adjust it.

Chapter 20

Step 3 – The Bridge Days

Understanding When You Need a Bridge

Now that you understand your Baseline eating, we need to address what happens when your power drops so low that your Baseline feels impossible and chaos feels like it's on the horizon. This is where a Bridge Day comes in – and understanding when to use it could be the difference between temporary difficulty and complete derailment.

What Bridge Days Are For

This is the plan you follow when you feel you need to be reset, refreshed, and stabilized. When your power is 1–4, you switch from your Baseline to these Bridge Days. Bridge Days are not failures by any means – they are acts of pre-emptive damage control built on self-awareness. They serve several crucial functions.

When you're already struggling, trying to maintain your usual standards often leads to even more chaos. Bridge Days allow you to focus on not making things worse rather than trying to make things better by going to default extremes one way or the other.

- When your power is low, every decision can feel like it takes too much energy. Bridge Days eliminate unnecessary decisions so you can focus your limited resources on getting through the day.
- Instead of depleting yourself further, a Bridge Day plan includes specific actions designed to restore your capacity.
- By having a separate protocol for crisis times, you don't associate your Baseline with periods of struggle. Your Baseline remains your preferred way of eating rather than something you have to force yourself to do, regardless of circumstances.

Bridge Days: Guidelines

Bridge Day foods

These should meet specific criteria that prioritize psychological safety and power conservation . . .

- **Nothing that typically creates chaos for you:** Avoid any foods that you've identified as consistently problematic for your mental state around eating. This isn't the time to test your capabilities or try to include challenging foods. If chocolate usually leads to a binge, Bridge Days are not the time to see if you can have 'just a little'.

- **Maximum comfort with minimum guilt:** Choose foods that feel nurturing and satisfying without creating additional emotional drama. Think gentle, familiar, soothing options. These might be foods that remind you of being cared for, that feel like a warm hug, that don't require complex preparation or decision-making.
- **Easy to obtain and prepare:** Your power is low, so Bridge Day foods should require minimal decision-making and preparation. Have options ready in advance. This might mean having frozen meals you actually enjoy, simple combinations like toast and butter, or foods that can be prepared with minimal steps.
- **Blood-sugar stabilizing:** Focus on combinations that will help you feel physically stable rather than foods that might cause crashes or additional cravings. You want foods that provide steady energy rather than quick highs followed by crashes that make everything feel harder.
- **Psychologically neutral:** Bridge Day foods shouldn't feel like punishment (too restrictive) or like giving up (too chaotic). They should feel like caring for yourself. They're not 'good' or 'bad' foods – they're tools for getting through a difficult time.

The key is to identify these foods in advance, when your power is higher, so you don't have to make these decisions when you're struggling.

Bridge Day activities

These should be actions designed to increase your power rather than deplete it further. You don't want to embark on any ambitious self-improvement projects – just simple actions that reliably help you feel more like yourself . . .

- **Sleep and rest**: Give yourself permission to sleep more, nap if you need to, and rest without feeling guilty about productivity. Sleep is one of the fastest ways to restore power, but it's often the first thing we sacrifice when we're stressed.
- **Hydration**: Simple but effective – often when our power is low, we're also dehydrated, which makes everything feel harder. Keep water nearby and drink it regularly. Don't worry about fancy hydration goals; just drink more water than you usually would.

Places you source power from

These are activities, environments, or practices that reliably make you feel more like yourself:

- Listening to specific music
- Being in nature
- Calling someone who makes you feel grounded
- Putting down a boundary
- Or any activity that reminds you of your strength, capability, and value

Bridge Day optics

You're not committing to a workout – you're just putting the mat out. Sometimes that leads to doing some gentle movement, sometimes it doesn't. Either way, you've done something that aligns with taking care of yourself. The power is in the intention and the tiny action, not in the follow-through. The message is that you're still on a mission, you're still creating associations, and your body and mind are worth taking care of, in every possible tiny way.

Taking Decision-Making Out of the Equation

One of the biggest causes of depleted power is decision fatigue. Bridge Days are designed to eliminate as many decisions as possible . . .

- **Pre-planned food options**: You've already decided what you'll eat on Bridge Days.
- **Simple routines**: Basic self-care actions that don't require planning or complicated execution.
- **Predetermined activities**: A menu of power-increasing activities to choose from rather than having to figure out what might help. You're not deciding whether a bath or a walk would be better – you're choosing from a pre-approved list of things that reliably help.
- **Clear structures**: You know in advance what you do and don't do on Bridge Days. You prepared your Bridge plan intentionally and you trust it enough to hand yourself over to it, having anticipated this

moment would find you when the version of you that has your most meaningful goals in mind and knows you the best wrote the Bridge plan in the first place. You don't have to decide whether it's okay to skip the gym or order takeaway – these decisions have already been made.

Hitting Pause

You don't look for opportunities to challenge yourself when you've identified that you should be executing Bridge Days. Your progress is built on the unhelpful things you manage not to do despite wanting to:

- Your only job is getting through the day doing what you said you were going to do.
- You're powerful in having pre-empted and prepared for periods of powerlessness.
- You focus on basic self-care, comfort, and stability, which take priority over growth and challenge. This is about maintaining rather than improving.

Building Your Bridge

The most important thing about a Bridge Day is that you plan it when your power is high, not when you need it. This is like having a fire escape plan – you figure out the route *before* the building is on fire.

- Literal food options: Identify 10 meals/snacks/takeaways/types of restaurant that meet your Bridge Day criteria and make sure you always have the

ingredients or information available. Write them down. Put them where you can find them easily.
- Comfort activities: Create a menu of power-increasing activities you can choose from without having to think of them in the moment. Include things that work in different circumstances – some that require going out, some that can be done at home.
- Plan how to make your environment as supportive as possible: This might mean having certain playlists ready, keeping your space tidy enough to feel calmer, or writing off planned chores to watch a movie.

Returning to Baseline

The transition back to your Baseline should be gradual and based on genuine power improvement, not calendar dates or external pressure. Assess honestly: Is your power actually 5+ or are you just tired of being in Bridge Days? Sometimes we want to return to Baseline because Bridge Days feels like 'giving up', but premature return often leads to another blip.

Start simple. Return to the easiest elements of your Baseline first, before adding complexity. Maybe start with the meal planning or other preparatory elements before tackling the food situations. Ultimately you want this neutral space to help you avoid the 'final binge' thinking that pending deadlines, diets, and discomfort have brought you in the past.

Chapter 21

Step 4 – Building Your Flight Record

Learning and Unlearning

Now that you have your power assessment, Baseline, and Bridge Days, we need to address how you'll actually change the specific behaviors that have been keeping you trapped in food chaos. This is where Building Your Flight Record comes in – your detailed curriculum for developing evidence that you can be trusted around food.

You need a curriculum. You need a list of things you find hardest to do that take you further away from where you want to be. These are behaviors that make you feel powerless, that you wouldn't recommend to someone you love, that feel hurried, or that you wouldn't engage in if someone you respected could see you. They are the all-or-nothing behaviors that make no sense for weight loss and make you feel stupid and self-sabotaging.

Two Interconnected Tracks

Unlearning efforts are the habits you'd never have chosen for yourself – the ones that are responsible for you not feeling calm, controlled, and as if you can be sensible with food to manage your weight and choices. These are behaviors that make you feel powerless, that you wouldn't recommend to someone you love, that feel hurried, or that you wouldn't engage in if someone you respected could see you.

Learning efforts are directly linked to the unlearning. For each unlearning effort, you identify what you need to learn/practise/turn into a habit to make that unlearning effort easier.

Your unlearning list is the stuff that builds up over time and punctuates your day with reminders that you and your body matter. Your learning list is there to support your unlearning list. If you keep doing the things on your learning list, regardless of where your bigger missions are, you are more likely to get back on track quickly because of the associations you've made, and – more fundamentally – your learning list will build your power for you.

Your power at any point is the number of steps you are between wanting to do something impulsively that you'll regret, and actually doing it.

Why This System Works

The Flight Record system works because it addresses the core problem that sabotages all sustainable change: the all-or-nothing thinking that makes you abandon everything when you struggle with one thing.

In the past, you probably grouped all your healthy habits together under 'being good'. When one habit failed, you felt you'd failed at everything, which led you to abandon all healthy habits until your next 'fresh start'.

The Flight Record prevents this by:

- **Separating each habit individually**: You can be improving your record of drinking water while still working on your record of not eating while cooking. One doesn't depend on the other.
- **Focusing on evidence over perfection**: Each time you successfully handle a challenging situation, you're building evidence that you can trust yourself. This evidence accumulates regardless of whether you're perfect.
- **Making the abstract concrete**: Instead of vague goals like 'eat healthy', you have specific, measurable behaviors that you can practise until they become automatic.
- **Building mastery through repetition**: Everything gets easier when you do it in a row. The Flight Record ensures you're practising specific skills repeatedly until they become effortless.

Building Your Personal Curriculum

You should be asking yourself all day every day during your learning period: What do I need to unlearn? And what do I need to learn to unlearn it? That way, you're reconnecting with your body again – not through body meditation or mindful massage but by noticing the experiences, sensations around food, body weight, or indeed anything that makes the chatter go up and the food noise start and makes you doubt yourself.

Think about these specific moments that tend to derail your progress:

- The moments when you haven't been perfect and think you've 'blown it'.
- When you think you've been perfect but your jeans feel tight, making you feel guilty and want to eat on that guilt.
- Finding out you're going on holiday and wanting to restrict for control or binge for comfort, instead of staying on track with the healthy plan you've committed to.
- When you have a really difficult day during the adjustment period, and not eating chocolate because you're learning not to when stressed feels too much like the hundreds of times you weren't 'allowed' chocolate, triggering the psychological response to eat chocolate 'one last time'.

Remember that this is just the adjustment of change. For people who understand that point where eating nothing is more sustainable than eating most foods, the second choice that turns into the thirtieth choice is the problem. Thinking we've gained weight ultimately makes us gain more weight.

When you're at work three days after creating your Flight Record plan and it's 3pm on Thursday and you're reminded that every time you see a certain colleague in a meeting at this time, you feel compelled to throw in the gym plans, and forget the healthy dinner. You never used to think about it much, just blamed yourself for not being healthy the next day.

But now you hear it – sack off the gym and get takeaway tonight – and with it comes a feeling. A familiar feeling that comes every Thursday and leaves the meeting room with you. 'Everyone thinks I'm stupid,' all because this woman triggers you in that way. And now you know that when you think and feel that way, your power goes down and the automatic part of you gets louder and wants you to act in ways that feel impulsive. But you choose to act with intention. Once you learn not to act impulsively, you can trust your plan and believe in it, and buckle up for the soundtrack.

This is how you start recognizing the patterns that have been running your eating behaviors without you being aware of them. Instead of just feeling bad about making poor choices, you start understanding the emotional and psychological triggers that lead to those choices.

The Evidence Collection Process

Think about identifying specific moments when you typically feel powerless or your plans get derailed. Be as detailed as possible:
- What time of day does this usually happen?
- What emotional state are you in?

- What physical state are you in?
- What typically triggers this moment?
- What thoughts go through your head?
- What actions do you typically take?
- How do you feel afterwards?

These moments become the foundation for building your Flight Record. Each moment represents a specific behavior pattern that you can isolate, understand, and systematically change through practise.

What Do I Need to Do in a Row Until It's Easier?

The fundamental principle of the Flight Record is this: everything gets easier when you do it consistently. But most people never experience this ease because they give up before the habit becomes automatic.

This time, not only is your success not simply measured in basic things like weight, but you don't even know the many things it will be measured in yet.

You need to ask yourself some basic questions:
- What do I need to do in a row until it's easier?
- How can I get myself to keep doing it in a row?
- What gets in the way of me doing it in a row?
- How can I still carry on even when I haven't done it in a row?
- Can I accept that doing it in a row is the only way to get it done and make it easy?
- Can I accept that it's not until I make decisions in the

hardest psychological circumstances that I will truly feel I can trust myself and believe that the chatter will go away?

Building Tolerance for Internal Backlash

Now we need to understand what creates the internal resistance that sometimes makes it feel impossible to keep building your Flight Record. There are different types of internal backlash that correspond directly to the four types of food noise we identified earlier. Understanding these patterns helps you prepare for them, rather than being derailed by them.

Physical Hunger Backlash

Physical hunger food chat: *These cravings are unbearable. I must have picked the wrong plan. I'll go nuclear until I find the right one. When I'm physically hungry, I forget how much I want to lose weight and I'll make the worst choices, eat in ways and contexts I'm not happy with, like fast, in the car.* There are periods in the day when physical hunger can set in motion a chain of choices that is responsible for a lot of weight gain.

Anyone who eats large amounts of sugar and ultra-processed foods, and overeats to the point of discomfort, and binges in anticipation of the next diet, will go through a phase of physical withdrawal. This isn't a character flaw – it's your body adjusting to a different way of eating. The cravings are real, they're temporary, and they don't mean you've picked the wrong plan.

Emotional Craving Backlash

Emotional hunger food chat: *I can't get through this without food to help me change how I feel. I'll give in now and binge one last time, then I'll start again when this stressful stage passes. I can't believe I've let it get this far, where I'm upset and worried about not being able to eat and where I'm still no closer to liking my body than I was when I started. This whole thing feels like it's never going to get easier and the harder it gets to stay on track, the more deprived I feel when I try to follow any kind of rules with food.*

You've been using food to manage your emotions for so long that it feels like the only reliable coping mechanism you have. But food doesn't actually change difficult emotions – it just postpones them. Learning to tolerate emotional discomfort without immediately reaching for food is a skill that gets easier with practise.

Decision-Making Backlash

Decision-making food chat: *I literally don't know what to eat and thinking about it is a chore. I can't do the perfect thing so I'll do the worst possible thing. I stick to a routine for a period and then I'm bored of the same meals or I stop making efforts and, before you know it, I'm winging it all the time.*

Food planning and decision-making is boring for everyone. It's administrative work that requires mental energy. The difference is that people without a complicated relationship with food don't interpret this boredom as evidence that they're failing.

HOW DIETS MAKE US FAT

Shame-Spiralling Backlash

Shame-spiralling food chat: *I can't control myself, I'm greedy and weak and I can't believe how much I just ate. That was a fluke, I'll never manage this anyway. There's no point trying to get through this, it'll never get easier.*

The shame voice will try to convince you that any struggle means you're fundamentally flawed. But struggling while learning a new skill is normal. The shame spirals become less frequent and less intense as you build evidence that you can handle challenging situations.

When it's personal

Why do we have food chat in our heads? Now we know what it is, let's think about what it's there for and when it comes up. When is it there most? When is it there least? What does food chat do? It makes you doubt your choices. It makes you feel overwhelmed. It makes you not trust yourself. Feel confused by conflicting diet advice. Reminds you of failure and makes it personal.

All food chat is personal unless it's 'I'm hungry and I need to eat.' And when it gets personal it stops being something you do in a row until it's easy. That means you stop factoring in any difficulty because you blame yourself and think it should be easier already. You have to make it *not personal*.

The moment food chatter becomes about your character, your worth, your capability as a person, it stops being a practical challenge and becomes an emotional crisis. This is why a food choice that feels manageable one day can feel impossible the next – it's not about the food, it's about what the food choice means about you.

Learning to recognize when food chat has become personal allows you to step back and remember that you're simply practising a skill. Skills require repetition. Skills get easier with practise. Skills don't reflect your worth as a person.

How to Build Flight Records That Work

Instead of saying you will go to the gym for 55 minutes Monday, Wednesday, and Friday, say that you'll drive to the gym, pack/wash your gym kit, charge your AirPods, leave the house in Lycra three times. Doing that allows you to catch the moments when there's least internal and/or external resistance and meet them with preparation to create the perfect conditions for doing something hard – activating your all-or-nothing thinking while thinking you're simply doing something tiny and easy.

If you know that you will go to the gym if you have your gym kit in the car, then don't worry about writing 'go to gym', just write 'put gym kit visible in car every day'. If you're used to thinking you've blown it if you assign days to go to the gym and when Tuesday doesn't happen because life gets in the way you don't do the rest, then give yourself flexibility within clear guidelines. Create fewer opportunities for perceived failure, and more opportunities to still be and get back in the zone. The key is to identify the smallest action that reliably leads to the behavior you want. Don't commit to the full behavior – commit to the point of no return that makes the full behavior almost inevitable.

Point-of-No-Return Hacks

The unlearning list also helps you to stumble upon 'point-of-no-return hacks'. These are the things you do that put you in the zone. The work you do on your Bridge Days will include reviewing these and making sure you really focus on them as you go back into Baseline.

One of my clients did this really well. For a long time before we met, he had a whiteboard of tasks he wasn't completing: 45 minutes on Peloton, cook a healthy dinner from scratch for him and his partner, and apply for eight jobs.

After our first session, we used this hack as he was an all-or-nothing perfectionist too. We wiped the board and replaced it with 'Lycra in the morning, cut an onion, open indeed.com website.' These were his points of no return.

He could do them at any time in the day and he knew that with Lycra on, he'd get on that Peloton. Likewise, once an onion was cut, he was looking around for a feast to cook. And once indeed.com was open, he wasn't closing his laptop. The tasks on the whiteboard were totally doable. And, of course, he did longer on the Peloton, and made better meals, and sent in better applications than before. Because he allowed himself the flexibility of all day not to feel like a failure, he found opportunities to take that one step to the point of no return, and trust that his all-or-nothing brain would take care of the rest.

My Point of No Return

I was never someone who felt compelled to exercise because I'd just eaten something unhealthy. At times when I was eating unhealthily, everything from bloating to acid reflux to the fact I'd never stuck with it long enough for it to be anything other than agony, was enough to make me only associate exercise with periods when I had already lost a lot of weight. Those were the times when I wanted to go to places like gyms because I didn't hate how I looked there, and I wanted to 'tone up'.

One Saturday morning, I'd forgotten that I'd made a plan with a friend to attend an (expensive) spin class at midday. I wouldn't get my money back and I'd be letting my friend down if I didn't show up. The problem was, the night before I'd broken yet another diet, and binged into the middle of the night, and by the time the reminder for my class popped up on my phone, I'd already had two very indulgent breakfasts.

From the moment I started bingeing on Friday night and planning what I'd eat, and what plans I'd cancel for the rest of the time period, I had no intention of doing anything healthy or social and certainly not weight-loss related until Monday morning. Since the beginning of my dieting journey as a child, a Friday night blow-out had always meant a write-off weekend of spiralling, bingeing, self-loathing, and eating everything I'd missed and would now never eat again 'one last time'. After all, you can't start again on Saturday.

This time, I went to the class. I felt horrible. I thought I was going to be sick. But then, by 1pm that Saturday, something happened by accident and I came upon a hack that I'd go on to share with countless clients. An all-or-nothing person who expects perfection (and so for that and other reasons is used to feeling a failure) needs to feel that they are doing well, that they're on a clear, existing mission, that they've been 'good'. That's what we thrive on. That's why when we see the scales go up, we respond to the disappointment of not losing weight by doing things that cause us to gain more.

If we had trick scales that told us we'd lost weight when we'd gained it, we'd be more likely to stay on track because we'd 'been good'; at least for a while anyway. Because we'd probably restrict out of over-excitement to speed it up and that would backfire into a binge.

And so, when I came out of the class, I didn't want to continue eating unhealthily. I associated excrcise with a huge investment in being in the zone, and the feeling of having done exercise and being in an exercise space and — even though it was horrible — not regretting it had an immediate domino effect because I associate it with weight loss. Exercise is something I normally only do when I'm already successful and unfortunately in my case that had always meant 'thin'. This time I wasn't thin, I was stuffed and withdrawing post-binge, and yet the whole thing turned around after one 45-minute class.

When I realized this, I started to reflect on my (often apparently absurd, irrelevant, and illogical) associations and find other things I could do to interrupt a spiral or binge to bring things back quickly. Often just deep breathing for two minutes would do it, once I got on board with the spirit of pattern interruption and redirection behind the hack.

Ask yourself: What would I never binge after doing? What could break the cycle of powerlessness earlier? What could turn Friday blips from Monday restarts to Saturday ones? And if you're chasing power and strength and collecting evidence for trust that brings mental quiet, then the kind choice is to 'go through the motions of behaving as though you're on track' by doing something you'd only do if you were on track, and then letting the rest of your habits take care of themselves.

Separating Your Flight Records to Prevent All-or-Nothing Thinking

When we chase results by repeating and making easier the choices that enable us to be happy with how we look and what we weigh, we have to separate all the new habits we're building. This way, you can go to bed thinking that the challenge of not comfort-eating after work hasn't seen a consistent record, but the challenges of not eating mindlessly in your car, making three healthy meals you enjoy per period, and not throwing in the towel after a choice that made you feel guilty are very much in play. You can watch yourself getting better at different things and see the long-term process more clearly.

While you build your Flight Record, you're building self-belief in the most important part: that you have the power to do anything in a row until it becomes easier. You have a process that factors in difficulty, discomfort, and adjustment. You've anticipated the internal and external backlash during adjustment and decided to treat it like any other habit change.

When your self-esteem has been attached to short-lived extreme measures, you'll find that building habits signalling that your body matters throughout the day – habits you would choose just to be a healthy human – insulates you when you do eat unhealthy foods in the future. Even if you hear old feelings of guilt, you're protected by automatic actions (like reaching for water) that remind you that you're someone who deserves care.

The Formula: One Choice After Another in a Row Until It's Easier

All you ever have to do is make the next best choice. All habit change is one choice in a row until it's easier. And choices come from chatter – internal chatter, food chatter, confusion, legacy thinking (it's a fluke), weight-loss thoughts, self-doubt, memories of failure, low self-belief, making food worse because you've made weight worse, all-or-nothing commands.

Clients often tell me they wish I could be in their pockets and keep repeating the things I remind them of during sessions, because it makes sense and they come away not doubting for a second why they're finding it hard, what process needs to take place for them to change (what they need to learn/unlearn), and why each new choice they need to make (however difficult) is not only possible, but also easier than countless other things they've done and achieved. The hard bit is believing that it's worth staying on track, believing in your capacity for mastery, believing in your plan of action for your hands, before your chatter and cravings get on board – *in order* to make them come on board and quieten down.

Flight Records Versus Food Chatter

By the time you have silenced the unhelpful food chat and regained control, you'll have learned and honed the most important aspect, not only of keeping up your results but also of creating plans for the rest of your life that are designed for your all-or-nothing mind, taking into account your personal history.

What if I told you that you're 50 challenges away from this being easy because you've built enough evidence? If you could do it once, you can do it over and over again. If you lose that logic, it gets personal and you forget that you need to do it in a row.

If you keep going with the learning list (even if the unlearning list isn't moving as fast), you'll see how it supports your unlearning efforts. Eventually these skills transfer: when you want to change any behavior – whether it's drinking wine, scrolling social media, or any other automatic response – you'll use the same process to reclaim your power.

The Grouping Effect: When It Clicks

When people start following this process, they'll ask questions like: *Will I have to practise this with every single food? What if I don't come across it for a while? What if this takes ages and my Flight Record is endless?*

I always tell them what I know to be true personally, and what I've seen to be true time and time again, every time a reader or coaching client tells me 'it just clicked.' What they're describing is a moment, or a period of time, when you realize that you're now just grouping foods into ones that turn up the chatter when your power is low, and ones that don't.

And you probably group apps the same way, come to think of it. The ones that take more than they give. In the same way I don't need to decide whether X is worse than Instagram for me right before I go to sleep; I just don't take my phone to bed because all the apps are grouped into a choice that I know I'll be tempted to make, a habit I know I'll be tempted to trivialize, and for that reason one that will be even easier to slip back into insidiously. Scrolling through phone apps is something I'm never ever glad I did, something I don't need an expert to tell me is bad for me, something that even if I don't know what's good for me, I know no one would recommend just before bed.

And so it goes, grouping foods and eating experiences based on what they do to your body and mind and what you notice. And the longer you stay on track, the more natural it becomes to keep up the habit of doing things that remind you that you do care about your body and mind (learning efforts), the more natural it feels to eat in ways you're proud of spontaneously and without much thought, and also to consume and let your body and mind be exposed to fewer things that take more than they give.

The 'click' moment is when these food choices become intuitive rather than effortful, when you naturally gravitate towards things that serve you and naturally avoid things that don't, without having to negotiate with yourself every time.

Chapter 22

Step 5 – Reclaiming Your Hands

Maintaining Agency in Crisis

This step is about reclaiming your hands – literally and metaphorically – from the feeling of being 'possessed' or 'out of control' when it comes to food. It's about proving to yourself that even when you're making choices you'd rather not make, you still have power and you're still in charge.

Understanding the Powerlessness Trap

One of the most damaging aspects of having a complicated relationship with food is the feeling that you become powerless around food – that your hands move without your permission, that you're 'possessed' by cravings, that something else takes over and makes choices for you.

This sense of powerlessness is what keeps people trapped

in shame cycles. When you feel you had no choice in what happened, you can't learn from the experience or build confidence for next time. Instead, you feel like a victim of your own impulses, which creates more shame, which drives more impulsive eating, which reinforces the sense of powerlessness.

But here's the truth: you are never actually powerless. Even when you're making choices you regret, even when you're eating in ways that don't serve you, even when you feel completely out of control – your hands are still your hands. You are still making choices, even if they don't feel conscious in the moment.

'Reclaiming your hands' is about acknowledging this truth and using it to maintain your sense of agency even in difficult moments.

Why This Matters for Your Recovery

Maintaining agency during difficult moments is crucial for several reasons . . .

- **It prevents shame spirals**: When you acknowledge that you chose to eat something, rather than feeling like it 'happened to you', you maintain your sense of control and self-respect. This avoids the shame spiral that often leads to more impulsive eating.
- **It enables learning**: When you *own* your choices, you can examine what led to them and make different choices next time. When you feel powerless, there's nothing to learn because 'it wasn't really you' making the decision.

- **It builds self-trust**: Each time you acknowledge your agency, even during difficult moments, you're proving to yourself that you're always in control. This builds confidence and self-trust over time.
- **It makes you the boss**: Feeling out of control around your choices can create a powerless mentality that keeps you stuck. Reclaiming agency puts you back in the driver's seat of your own life.

The Practice of Getting in Front of It

If you find yourself in the middle of a blow-out, totally out of control, and it's likely that at some point in life you will do again, then there is one thing you can absolutely do. You can decide to get in front of it and simply acknowledge what you're doing and that you're choosing to do it. That's it. Even in that moment where everything feels hurried again and you're trying to eat as much as you can, before the disappointment of what you're doing hits you, knowing when it does you will eat even more. Even when you've gained weight and you feel like nothing has changed, there is a way to claim back all the self-knowledge and fundamental power you know you have. And that is simply to *own* what you are doing.

This practice may seem simple but it's incredibly powerful. In the moment when you feel most out of control, you pause and say to yourself: 'I am choosing to eat this. There are reasons why I'm making this choice. My hands are my hands.'

This isn't about stopping the behavior or making yourself feel guilty about it. It's about reclaiming your agency and preventing the experience from reinforcing feelings of powerlessness.

What This Sounds Like in Practice

Here are a few examples of how to reclaim your hands in different situations:

- **During a binge**: 'I am choosing to keep eating these biscuits. I'm feeling overwhelmed and this is how I'm coping right now. This is my choice.'
- **When eating emotionally**: 'I am choosing to eat this chocolate because I'm stressed about work. Food feels like the easiest way to manage this feeling right now.'
- **When making impulsive choices**: 'I am choosing to order takeaway instead of cooking. I'm tired and this feels easier tonight.'

Notice that these statements don't include judgment or attempts to stop the behavior. They simply acknowledge that you are making conscious choices with your own hands for your own reasons.

Why This Isn't About Stopping Yourself

It's important to understand that reclaiming your hands isn't about developing the willpower to stop eating when you don't want to stop. It's not about using this awareness to control your behavior in the moment.

Trying to use this technique to control your eating will backfire because it turns reclaiming agency into another form of restriction. The power of this practice comes from the acknowledgment itself, not from changing what you do.

When you consistently practise acknowledging your choices without trying to change them, several things happen:

- **You stop feeling like a victim of your impulses**: You recognize that you always have reasons for your choices, even if those reasons don't always serve your long-term goals.
- **You maintain your sense of self**: Instead of feeling like 'someone else' took over during difficult eating moments, you maintain continuity of identity.
- **You gather information**: By acknowledging why you're making choices in the moment, you learn about your patterns and triggers without judgment.
- **You build confidence**: Each time you reclaim agency, you prove to yourself that you're capable of being conscious and aware even during challenging moments.

Unhealthy Choices: An Everybody Problem

People who haven't developed a complicated relationship with food make unhealthy choices too. For the rest of your life, you will make unhealthy choices. The point is to not make extremely unhealthy ones consistently and frequently and to choose the ones you're going to make. This perspective is crucial for reclaiming your hands. The goal isn't to become someone who never makes impulsive food choices or never eats for emotional reasons. The goal is to become someone who feels they can make those choices consciously, calmly, and intentionally.

When you see someone who doesn't have a complicated relationship with food eat an entire bag of crisps while watching a film, they don't spiral into shame or feel like they've lost control. They might think *I ate more than I intended* or *I'm quite full now* and then move on with their evening. They maintain their sense of agency throughout the experience.

The Power of 'I Am Choosing'

The phrase 'I am choosing' is incredibly powerful because it immediately shifts you from victim to agent. It acknowledges that:

- **You have reasons and you know them – and yourself**: Even choices that don't serve your long-term goals make sense in the moment, based on your emotional state, energy levels, circumstances, and coping mechanisms.
- **You have power – and sometimes you use it to rebel**: Your hands belong to you, your choices belong to you, and you are capable of making different choices when you're ready.
- **You are learning – and you don't need to be perfect**: Each choice provides information about what you need, what triggers you, and what serves you.

HOW DIETS MAKE US FAT

When Reclaiming Your Hands Feels Difficult

Sometimes acknowledging your choices will feel uncomfortable because it means taking responsibility for decisions you'd rather blame on something else. This discomfort is normal and part of the growth process.

If you find you are resisting the practice of reclaiming your hands, ask yourself:

- What am I afraid will happen if I acknowledge that I'm choosing this? Often the fear is that acknowledgment means you're 'bad' or that you'll have to stop. Neither is true.
- What would it mean about me if I admitted that I'm choosing this? If you're holding on to the belief that good people don't make impulsive food choices, acknowledging your choices challenges this belief.
- Am I trying to use this practice to control my behavior? If you're using awareness as a tool to stop eating, it won't work and will create resistance.

Remember that the power of reclaiming your hands comes from the acknowledgment itself, not from changing your behavior. Trust the process and be patient with yourself as you develop this skill.

Looking Ahead

Over time, consistently practising this skill creates profound changes in your relationship with food:

- **Reduced shame**: When you stop feeling like a victim of your impulses, shame around food choices naturally decreases.
- **Increased self-trust**: As you prove to yourself repeatedly that you're always in control, your confidence around food grows.
- **Better decision-making**: When you acknowledge your choices without judgment, you gather better information about what serves you and what doesn't.
- **Greater flexibility**: When you're not afraid of making imperfect choices, you can be more flexible and spontaneous around food.
- **Peace of mind**: When you know you can handle any food situation by maintaining your agency, food loses its power to create anxiety.

The practice of reclaiming your hands is simple but not always easy. It requires courage to take responsibility for your choices and compassion to do so without judgment. But it's one of the most powerful tools for transforming your relationship with food from one of powerlessness to one of empowered choice.

Chapter 23

Step 6 – Reclaiming Forbidden Territory

Strategic Approaches to Challenging Foods

Now that you've developed the skill of maintaining agency during difficult moments, we can address one of the most complex aspects of food recovery: working strategically with foods that feel challenging or trigger chaos.

By the time you're ready for this step, you should have evidence that you can handle your Baseline eating consistently, that you can navigate Bridge Days without complete chaos, that you can build your Flight Record, and that you can reclaim your hands during difficult moments. If you're not there yet, return to the chapters about building those foundational elements. Working with challenging foods without a solid foundation will feel overwhelming and set you back.

This step addresses the foods that don't fit neatly into

your Baseline – the ones that spike your food noise even when your power is on point, that test your Flight Record most severely, and make reclaiming your hands most crucial.

Understanding Challenging Foods Versus Trigger Foods

First, we need to distinguish between challenging foods and trigger foods, because they require completely different approaches.

Challenging foods require more mental bandwidth to handle calmly but don't automatically trigger chaos. They might be foods you love but tend to overeat, foods that bring up some guilt or food noise, or foods that you struggle to include in appropriate portions. With practise and the right circumstances, you can learn to include these foods in your Baseline.

Examples might include:
- Foods you enjoy but historically overeat (like nuts or chocolate)
- Foods that bring up diet mentality guilt (like bread or pasta)
- Foods that you struggle to eat in controlled portions
- Foods that feel 'too indulgent' but don't trigger complete chaos

Trigger foods consistently activate your shame-spiral noise, regardless of your power, circumstances, or intentions. These are foods where 'just one bite' reliably leads to eating the entire packet, where the guilt and chaos are so intense that they derail your eating for days, where the food noise becomes deafening. These foods may need to be excluded from your Baseline temporarily or permanently, and that's not a failure – it's strategic self-care.

Examples might include:
- Foods that you cannot have in the house without eating all of them
- Foods that trigger multi-day binges or complete loss of control
- Foods so loaded with shame that eating them derails your entire day
- Foods that activate such intense all-or-nothing thinking that recovery becomes impossible

The key difference is that challenging foods can become neutral with practise, while trigger foods may always require careful management or avoidance. Both approaches are valid, and the choice depends on your individual patterns and what serves your long-term wellbeing.

The Decision Framework: Include or Exclude?

For each food that feels problematic, you need to make a strategic decision: Will you work towards including this food in your life, or will you exclude it temporarily or permanently?

Diet culture tells you that you 'should' be able to include all foods, that excluding any food is restriction, and will lead to rebellion. But this ignores the reality that some foods may genuinely not serve some people, and that strategic exclusion can be an act of self-care rather than restriction.

Consider inclusion if:
- The food brings genuine pleasure and has positive associations
- You have evidence that you can sometimes handle it calmly
- The chaos it creates is manageable and doesn't last long
- You have strong emotional or cultural connections to the food
- Excluding it feels punitive rather than caring
- You believe you can develop skills to handle it better

Consider exclusion if:
- The food consistently triggers extended chaos regardless of circumstances
- The effort required to include it mindfully feels disproportionate to the benefit
- You have clear evidence that your life is better without this food
- Including it compromises other areas of your wellbeing
- The food is strongly linked to trauma or painful memories
- Exclusion feels empowering rather than restrictive

Remember: you can always change your mind. You might exclude a particular food temporarily while you build other skills, then revisit the decision later. Or you might try including a food, and then discover that exclusion serves you better.

The Process for Working with Challenging Foods

When you decide to work towards including challenging foods – and only when your Baseline feels secure and your power is consistently high – here's the strategic approach:

- **Start with foods that are mildly challenging,** not your biggest triggers. Choose foods that create some food noise but don't send you into complete chaos. Think of this as building your tolerance gradually, like training for a marathon by starting with shorter distances. You might start with a food that you enjoy but tend to overeat slightly, rather than jumping straight to the food that has historically triggered extended binges.
- **Create optimal conditions for success.** Plan to work with challenging foods when your power is high, you're in your own environment, you have no other stressors, and you have support available if needed. Don't attempt it when you're tired, stressed, or dealing with other difficulties. This might mean choosing a relaxed time when you're well-rested and calm, rather than when you're depleted from work.
- **Have a specific plan for the experience.** Decide in advance how much you'll have, in what context, and what you'll do afterwards. This isn't about restriction

– it's about creating structure that supports success. You might decide to have a small portion with a meal, or to buy a single serving, rather than a family-size packet.

- **The plan should feel caring rather than controlling.** You're setting yourself up for success, not imposing arbitrary rules.
- **Practise the skill of eating challenging foods within your Baseline.** The goal isn't to prove you can binge on challenging foods without any consequences – it's to prove you can include them in amounts and contexts that feel good and don't trigger chaos. This means eating them as part of meals, when you're appropriately hungry, in social contexts, or however feels most natural and sustainable.
- **Expect food noise and prepare for it.** Your automatic brain will likely protest when you introduce challenging foods. This is normal and expected. Have scripts ready for when the food noise gets loud: *This is just my brain being worried, I'm practising a skill, this feeling is temporary.* The noise might sound like: *You shouldn't be eating this, you're going to want more, this is going to trigger a binge, you can't be trusted.* Prepare your responses in advance.
- **Focus on the evidence you're building.** Each time you successfully navigate a challenging food situation, you're proving to yourself that you can be trusted. This evidence accumulates and makes future encounters easier.

- **Don't dismiss successes as 'flukes.'** Each positive experience with a challenging food is further proof that you can handle these situations.
- **Don't rush the process.** There's no timeline for when challenging foods should become neutral. Some foods might require extended practise. Some foods might never become Baseline foods, and that's acceptable. Rushing the process often leads to overwhelm and setbacks. Trust that skills develop over time with consistent practise.

Bringing Back Chocolate

Here's how this worked with chocolate for me. For an extended period, chocolate was a complete trigger food. I couldn't have it in the house without eating all of it. The guilt and shame around chocolate were so intense that even thinking about having it would trigger a binge-restriction cycle.

When I was ready to work with chocolate – after my Baseline felt secure and I had evidence that I could trust myself in other food situations – I started very small. I began by having a small piece of good-quality chocolate after dinner when I was already satisfied, in my own home, with nothing else stressful happening.

The food noise was loud at first: *You shouldn't be eating this, you're going to want more, this is going to trigger a binge*. But I had prepared for this noise. I reminded myself that I was practising a skill, that the noise was my automatic brain being worried, and that the feeling was temporary.

I practised this scenario many times – having a small piece of chocolate after dinner and then stopping. Not because I was restricting myself, but because that's what I had planned and it felt good. Gradually, the food noise around chocolate got quieter. It became just another food that I could include or not include, based on what I wanted and what served me.

Now chocolate is a neutral food for me. I can have it or not have it. I can buy it and forget it's in the cupboard. I can have a small amount or sometimes choose to have more, and either choice feels calm and intentional rather than chaotic.

This didn't happen quickly, and it didn't happen by forcing myself to have chocolate when I wasn't ready. It happened by building my skills gradually and only working with chocolate when I had the bandwidth to handle whatever came up.

Working with Food Environments

Part of reclaiming forbidden territory involves learning to exist peacefully in environments where challenging or excluded foods are present. You need to be able to go to parties, restaurants, and social gatherings without feeling anxious or deprived.

For challenging foods you're working to include:
- Practise being around these foods without eating them sometimes
- Practise having small amounts in social situations
- Practise returning to your Baseline after including them

For foods you've chosen to exclude:
- Practise being around excluded foods without feeling deprived
- Develop scripts for declining these foods gracefully
- Focus on what you can enjoy rather than what you're not having
- Remember that your choice to exclude is valid and caring

The Social Aspect of Challenging Foods

Many challenging foods are also social foods – birthday cake, holiday treats, foods that are central to cultural or family traditions. This adds further complexity because you're not just managing your individual relationship with the food, but also navigating social expectations and relationships.

Strategies for social food situations:
- Decide your approach before attending events
- Have phrases ready for declining foods gracefully
- Focus on the social aspects rather than the food
- Bring alternatives if appropriate
- Practise flexibility within your boundaries
- Remember that other people are usually much less focused on your food choices than you think

Building Food Neutrality Over Time

The ultimate goal of working with challenging foods is food neutrality – the ability to make calm, rational decisions about all foods based on your circumstances, preferences, and what serves your wellbeing.

Food neutrality doesn't mean you like all foods equally or that all foods serve you equally. It means that your food choices are based on practical considerations rather than emotional reactivity.

Signs of food neutrality:
- You can be around any food without anxiety
- Your food choices are based on preference and circumstances rather than rules
- You don't feel guilty about eating any particular food
- You don't feel deprived when you choose not to eat something
- Food decisions feel as neutral as other daily choices
- You trust yourself to make appropriate choices in any situation

The Forbidden Territory Paradox

There's a paradox in reclaiming forbidden territory: the more peace you make with challenging foods, the less you may actually want them. When foods lose their 'forbidden' quality, they often lose their appeal as well.

This happens because much of the desire for forbidden foods comes from the restriction and rebellion cycle. When foods are no longer forbidden, when you know you can have them whenever you want them, the urgency and craving often diminish naturally.

Don't be surprised if foods you used to obsess over

become genuinely uninteresting once you've resolved the psychological drama around them. This is a sign of success, not deprivation.

Maintenance and Evolution

Your relationship with challenging foods will continue to evolve throughout your life. Foods that feel challenging now may become neutral later. Foods that you exclude temporarily may become includable. Foods that you include now may become problematic during stressful life periods.

This evolution is normal and doesn't represent failure or regression. Your food choices should serve your current life circumstances and wellbeing, not some fixed ideal of what a 'recovered' person should eat. Stay curious about your relationships with different foods, and be willing to adjust your approach based on what you learn about yourself over time. The goal is a flexible, sustainable relationship with food that serves your overall wellbeing, not rigid adherence to any particular eating philosophy.

Remember: you are reclaiming territory that was never actually forbidden. These are just foods, and you are a capable adult who can make wise choices about what serves you. The forbidden territory was created by diet culture's rules and restrictions. As you reclaim it, you're not just changing your relationship with specific foods – you're reclaiming your autonomy and trust in yourself.

Chapter 24

Step 7 – Changing Your Internal Script

Understanding the Internal Conflict

It's time to address the internal voice that will either support or sabotage all your efforts. This might be the most important step in this entire framework, because all the tools in the world won't help if your internal dialogue undermines your progress.

Food chatter is evidence that you've gone back into the automatic brain part of yourself. It's an alert that something has happened. Forgetting that you can choose what you want, and that food isn't more powerful than you are, is a call to action that we should be grateful for.

When food chatter goes up after the adjustment and self-awareness periods have passed, it's sounding an alarm. Comfort, control, old ways, forgetting we are smart and capable, forgetting about mastery, forgetting to zoom out – that automatic bit will try to hang on and the chatter it gives you isn't there to bring up the past and make you feel terrible; it's there because it's worried about you. It's worried that you'll suffer; it doesn't know what's next and it only has the past to go on.

This automatic brain doesn't know about a healthier you being better. It's operating from a locked-in-time place, developmentally and emotionally arrested, behaving the way it always has, ever since the first time hunger was imposed on it without it understanding why but knowing it was because there was something wrong with them and that all of a sudden food became something bad that would be taken away.

This automatic part has watched you try to starve yourself repeatedly. It's watched you get hurt and disappointed and ill and confused and jittery every time you go overboard with diets. It's seen the struggles you attempt to put up with after you eat a lot, and it's scared that one day you'll succeed at starving yourself for as long as you want to. It tells you what you need to hear so that you don't succeed. It's saying *Hey, you shouldn't/can't/do this, this isn't for you, you don't want to do this, you've never done it before* . . . not to be mean, but because it really doesn't want you to manage to starve yourself.

The Protective Function of Food Chatter

Understanding this protective function completely changes how you relate to your internal dialogue. Instead of seeing food chatter as evidence that you're broken or lacking willpower, you can recognize it as a protective mechanism that's trying to keep you safe based on outdated information.

Your automatic brain has watched you hurt yourself through dieting repeatedly. It has learned that attempts to change your eating always lead to restriction, deprivation, eventual loss of control, and shame. From the automatic brain's perspective, any attempt to change eating patterns is a threat to survival.

It doesn't care about evidence showing that sustainable approaches work. It doesn't care about your rational understanding of why this time is different. It only cares about the pattern it has observed: food changes = threat and suffering. So it will do everything in its power to prevent you from succeeding at changing your eating patterns.

This is why your internal dialogue often becomes most critical and sabotaging when you're actually making progress. It's not evidence that you're failing – it's evidence that your automatic brain is worried you might succeed at something it believes will hurt you.

Making It Impersonal

Getting rid of food chatter is about bringing that part up to date, to the age you are today. By showing it can come out unscathed. By soothing it but expecting it to put up a fight. By showing it that it doesn't have to keep you protected anymore. But you have to *show it*. You can't just tell it. And you have to get ready for it to push back against you. In fact, you have to thank it for pushing against you – it's done what evolution meant it to do.

This is crucial to understand: you cannot reason your way out of food chatter. You cannot convince your automatic brain with rational arguments. That part has heard all the reasonable explanations about why this time will be different. What it needs is proof, through your actions, that you can be trusted to take care of both parts of yourself.

The goal isn't to eliminate food chatter entirely – it's to make it impersonal. Food chatter doesn't disappear – it becomes predictable, impersonal, boring. It becomes noise uninformed by the mistrust that linking eating and weight loss created.

When food chatter becomes impersonal, you can hear it without being controlled by it. You'll notice the thought *I shouldn't eat this* without feeling compelled to either eat it rebelliously or avoid it restrictively. It becomes background noise, rather than a command you must obey.

Self-Compassion as Strategy

Assume that you will want extremes. I have good news for you. There is one area in which this approach allows you to live in the extremes and that is self-care and self-compassion. At times when you feel that you've let yourself down or your power is low, as we've said before, I don't want you to quickly revert to control or comfort and try to change how you look or feel with food or exercise. But what will always help is practising self-compassion.

Firstly, outside of your food choices, what are the things you do for yourself when you're on a health mission that are to do with general wellbeing? Do you meditate? Do you listen to nice music? Do you take more care of your appearance?

Secondly, what are the self-care acts that you take part in only when you're happy with the way your body looks, or you're on the way to improving your health and feeling excited? These can include things like taking pride in your appearance, hanging out with your friends, moisturizing, using that nice candle you've been saving for when you feel better about yourself, wearing those soft socks.

When I talk about self-care and self-compassion, I'm still thinking about it in the context of impulse control, getting back on track, getting the train back in the station, and you feeling calm and good. I'm also talking about things that pre-emptively increase your power, regardless of how you feel naturally and regardless of the strategies but as a foundational investment into feeling generally more robust physically and mentally.

When it comes to self-compassion and self-care exercises, there is no maximum that you can do. It's at times when you feel less deserving of self-kindness that you should be giving it most. You are allowed to forgive yourself quickly, you are allowed to be kind to yourself and speak kindly to yourself. I know it feels silly, but you are.

When we behave in a particular way towards other people, they are involved in how kind we can be to ourselves, based on their reaction. But when it comes to self-kindness, you are in charge of your reaction to the kindness levels that you show yourself. You are allowed to get something wrong and treat yourself the way you would treat a friend who you knew didn't deserve to beat themselves up, despite having done something wrong that had the potential to derail them in some way. Even if you were protecting them from what they had done, you would know that it was harmless to do so. That's the degree of support and backing I want you to allow yourself to give yourself.

Self-Compassion Requires Perspective

Self-compassion also requires perspective – zooming out. The famous Cher quote 'if it doesn't matter in five years it doesn't matter' comes to mind. It's extremely important for you to balance taking this whole exercise seriously (because of the damage that's been done to your mind, body, and quality of life) while also acknowledging the triviality and silliness of the fact that we're actually only talking about food.

Most of the things you beat yourself up about regarding your food choices will be completely irrelevant in a few years. The shame you carry about eating a packet of biscuits last Tuesday has no bearing on your long-term wellbeing. But the pattern of shaming yourself for normal human behavior will impact every day of your life until you change it.

This perspective isn't about minimizing your goals or saying food choices don't matter – it's about giving individual decisions the correct emotional weight. When you can zoom out and see the bigger picture, individual food choices become much less loaded with meaning about your character, worth, or future success. A challenging eating day becomes just that – one day – rather than evidence that you're fundamentally flawed.

The Mourning Process: Losing Food Noise

By the way, there is also an element of mourning involved in losing food noise. Some food noise is about planning and getting excited and distracting yourself from bigger problems by perfectly planning a diet. Other food noise involves getting excited about eating things that you find delicious. The problem gets even more complicated when we accept that one of the ways we keep trying to cut food noise is by eating food – in other words, the way we plan to change any unpleasant feeling.

This is important to acknowledge: food has been serving multiple functions in your life beyond nutrition. It's provided entertainment, comfort, distraction, rebellion, control, and reward. When food noise quiets, you might initially feel bored or empty because you've lost a major source of mental stimulation.

Your new internal script needs to help you through this transition by acknowledging the loss while focusing on what you're gaining: mental space, emotional freedom, trust in yourself, and the ability to use food for nourishment and genuine pleasure rather than emotional management.

The mourning process is normal and temporary. Many people are surprised by how much mental space they have once food noise quiets. Initially this can feel uncomfortable because you're used to having food thoughts occupy so much of your mental bandwidth.

Your internal script during this period should sound supportive: *It's normal to feel strange when food noise quiets. I'm learning to use my mental energy in new ways. This empty feeling is temporary as I adjust to food freedom.*

Reclaiming Your Hands: Agency in Crisis

One of the most important functions of your new internal script is supporting you in reclaiming agency during difficult moments, as we mentioned earlier.

The next time you find yourself eating in ways you don't want, you need to get in front of it. It's enough to say 'I am choosing to do this and there are reasons why I'm choosing to do this.' But I also want you to be able to reclaim your hands even when they are doing things that you are generally trying not to do any more. You need to remember that this is just your hands playing out and your body playing up, one of those blips that occur in the process of mastering something. But the most important thing is not to lapse back into the thought that you are powerless. That is the true relapse. Actions are just things that need to be done in an order until they become easy.

Your internal script should support this practice by offering phrases like:
- 'I am choosing this. There are reasons for my choice.'
- 'My hands belong to me. I am in control even when making choices I regret.'

- 'This is a blip in the process of learning, not evidence that I'm powerless.'
- 'I can reclaim my agency at any moment.'
- 'Making imperfect choices doesn't mean I'm out of control.'

This practice of reclaiming agency even during difficult moments is crucial if you are going to maintain your sense of power and control. It prevents the victim mentality that keeps you stuck in cycles of guilt and rebellion.

The Interview with Your Future Self

Imagine if you woke tomorrow at your goal size, with headspace about food, and raised confidence levels. You got there. And now it's easy to stay there, not because you've changed who you are but because you've managed to stay on track and keep gathering evidence until the habits that help you keep weight off feel automatic. In addition, the strategies you used to stay on track when your power was low or you weren't perfect or you had a setback are no longer strategies. They have now become your status quo – your default way of living.

I want you to imagine that you're being interviewed about your journey. About what you had to go through, prove to yourself, experience and overcome in order to truly trust yourself around food. About what made this time different and what choices you made to stay on track when it was hardest. I want you to imagine you're sitting there, proud, calm and completely informed and wise and reasonable when it comes to yourself as well as the process of change and mastery.

This visualization exercise helps your internal script start speaking from a place of success rather than fear. Instead of constantly preparing for failure, you start preparing for success.

Understanding Fluke Thinking

You need to accept that your food choices, once separated from each other and treated like any other skill you are building, will get easier once you have gathered evidence. The evidence gathering is to calm your body, help you come out unscathed, and build proof that's harder to push back against.

But it's also not actually required. If you accept that your changes will come down to one choice in a row in the end, no matter how many choices you need to unlearn/learn/practise, and you accept that each of those choices are doable, and that in a row they will become automatic, then you can remind yourself every single time that you believe in the plan and this formula, and this problem can be over *today*. In the end this is all about proving to yourself what you already know and what is evident when anyone looks at you.

Then of course you have to deal with the backlash of thinking that it was a fluke. Which of course should be one of the things that you expect. Fluke thinking is one of the most common ways your internal critic undermines success.

Every time you make a good choice, handle a challenging situation well, or stick to your plan when it's difficult, the fluke voice says: *That was just lucky, it won't last, don't get too confident.*

Your new internal script needs to be prepared for these comments and have responses ready:
- 'I've been building skills systematically, this isn't luck.'
- 'Each success builds on the previous ones.'
- 'I expected this to feel uncertain at first.'
- 'Dismissing my progress doesn't protect me, it undermines me.'
- 'Fluke thinking is just my automatic brain being worried.'
- 'I'm gathering evidence of my capability one choice at a time.'

The Next Best Choice

All habit change is one choice in a row until it's easier. And choices come from chatter – internal chatter, food chatter, confusion, legacy thinking (it's a fluke), weight-loss thoughts, self-doubt, memories of failure, low self-belief, making food worse because you've made weight worse, all-or-nothing commands.

Your internal script needs to consistently remind you that:
- Your body's signals are information, not sabotage
- Hunger and cravings are normal biological functions
- The difficulty you experience is evidence of learning, not failing

- Every choice is an opportunity to build evidence of your capability
- You have the power to make the next best choice regardless of what happened before

Developing Your Internal Coach Voice

Your internal coach should sound like you at maximum power supporting a friend. They:
- Believe in your capability unconditionally
- View difficulty as an expected part of learning, not evidence of failure
- Respond to setbacks with curiosity rather than criticism
- Alway help you focus on the next right choice rather than dwelling on past mistakes
- Treat food challenges like any other skill that requires practise
- Remind you that everything you're experiencing is normal and temporary
- Celebrate progress without dismissing it as a fluke
- Maintain perspective about the long-term journey

The Power Assessment and Internal Dialogue

We can use power daily to identify where we're at and what we need, reframing challenges as opportunities and putting strategies in place if we need to. But it's important to be aware of one thing that can trip us up – and that is that sometimes it will feel as though your power is high because you're losing weight, and you may have underestimated the extent to which that fact in itself is what's making you think your power is high.

So how do you know whether your power is high for a reason that will backfire on you, like this one, because you've attached food and weight again? And how do you know if your power is legitimately high? The answer is to think about your body and where that's at, rather than simply where the food chat is at. When you say you have more energy, do you mean in spirits for the day or a genuine sustained greater energy? How frequently are you hungry? How likely would you be to keep this up on your worst day?

Your internal script needs to help you distinguish between real confidence based on skill-building, and artificial confidence based on weight-loss excitement. Real confidence feels steady and grounded. Artificial confidence feels brittle and dependent on external validation.

Questions your internal script should ask:
- 'Is this confidence coming from skills I've built or from numbers on a scales?'
- 'Would I feel this capable if my weight had fluctuated upwards this period?'
- 'Am I assessing my power based on genuine resources or temporary excitement?'
- 'What evidence do I have of my capability beyond weight changes?'

Scripts for Common Challenging Moments

Here are some examples of how your new internal script should sound in common challenging situations:

- **When you make a choice you regret:** *I made a choice that didn't serve me. This is information about what I need or what triggered me. What can I learn from this? What's my next best choice?*
- **When you feel like you're not making progress fast enough:** *Skills develop at their own pace. I'm building evidence of my capability every day, even when I can't see it. Progress isn't always linear or visible.*
- **When you encounter a trigger food:** *This is an opportunity to practise a skill. I can choose what serves me right now. Whatever I choose, I can reclaim my hands and make the next choice consciously.*
- **When you're doing Bridge Days (or Weeks!):** *I'm being strategic about my resources right now. This is self-care, not giving up. I'll return to my Baseline when I'm ready.*
- **When old patterns resurface:** *Old patterns are familiar, not permanent. I'm in the process of building new patterns. Every time I notice and redirect is evidence of my growing awareness.*
- **When someone comments on your eating or weight:** *Other people's opinions about my food choices don't define my worth or determine my decisions. I trust myself to know what serves me.*

HOW DIETS MAKE US FAT

The goal here is to help you develop an internal voice that supports your success. This means:
- Understanding that the automatic brain is trying to protect you, based on old information about dieting and restriction being dangerous
- Learning to thank and reassure that part of yourself while still moving forwards with your reflective brain's knowledge and plans
- Practising extreme self-compassion especially during moments when you feel you're failing or struggling
- Reclaiming your agency even during difficult moments by acknowledging your choices rather than feeling powerless
- Making the process impersonal by treating food challenges like any other skill that requires practise
- Building evidence slowly and consistently that you can handle increasingly challenging situations around food.

The internal script you're developing should sound like someone who believes in your capability, expects difficulty as part of learning, responds to setbacks with curiosity rather than criticism, and always helps you focus on the next right choice rather than dwelling on past mistakes.

It becomes the voice that guides you back to your Baseline after Bridge Days, helps you choose appropriate challenges when your power is high, and reminds you that everything you're experiencing is part of the normal process of developing mastery around food.

Chapter 25

Step 8 – Emotional Regulation Without Food

Understanding Emotional Eating Versus Emotional Regulation

Now that you've developed a supportive internal script, we need to address one of the most challenging aspects of food recovery: learning to withstand difficult emotions without automatically reaching for food (when we know it can change how we feel in an instant).

Most approaches to emotional eating focus on identifying triggers and finding alternative activities – go for a walk instead of eating ice cream, call a friend instead of ordering takeaway. While these strategies can be helpful, they miss the deeper issue: most people who eat emotionally never actually learned how to process emotions in the first place.

The problem isn't that you use food to cope with emotions. The problem is that you never learned that emotions are temporary experiences that you can tolerate and process without needing to change them immediately. Food became your primary emotional regulation tool because it works quickly and reliably. It always changes how you feel, at least temporarily.

You eat to numb anxiety, comfort sadness, celebrate joy, or manage stress. The food is medicating the emotion rather than allowing you to experience and process it. Emotional regulation is the ability to experience emotions without being overwhelmed by them or needing to change them immediately. It means understanding that emotions are temporary, that you can tolerate discomfort, and that feelings provide information rather than emergencies that must be fixed.

The goal isn't to eliminate emotional eating entirely – people who haven't developed complicated relationships with food sometimes eat for emotional reasons too. The goal is to develop enough emotional regulation skills that food becomes one choice among many, rather than your automatic response to any difficult feeling.

Building Tolerance for Emotional Discomfort

The foundation of emotional regulation is building tolerance for uncomfortable feelings . . .

- **Even the most intense feelings peak and then subside naturally**: If you don't interfere with the process, the urge to eat emotionally often passes if you can tolerate the discomfort for a brief period.

- **Emotions provide information**: Feelings tell you about your needs, values, and circumstances. Anxiety might indicate that you need more support or preparation. Sadness might indicate that you need connection or grieving time. Anger might indicate that your boundaries have been violated.
- **Emotions don't require immediate action**: You can feel anxious without needing to eliminate the anxiety immediately. You can feel sad without needing to cheer yourself up right away. You can feel angry without needing to suppress it or act on it immediately.
- **You are bigger than your emotions**: You can experience intense feelings without being overwhelmed by them. Emotions are experiences you have, not who you are.
- **Building this tolerance requires practise**: Start with small, manageable emotional experiences and gradually work up to more challenging ones.

Instead of relying solely on food for emotional regulation, you need to develop a toolkit of strategies that work for different emotions and circumstances.

Exercise 1: Building Your Emotional Regulation Toolkit

For the next few days, notice when you eat emotionally and identify which category it falls into:
- Comfort eating (soothing negative emotions). Think about: What makes you feel cared for? What creates

physical warmth or softness? What helps you feel safe? What would you do for a friend who felt this way?
- Stress eating (managing anxiety/overwhelm). Think about: What helps you feel grounded? What releases physical tension? What gives you a sense of control? What helps you breathe easier?
- Reward eating (celebrating or treating yourself). Think about: What makes you feel special? What feels indulgent without food? What would you do to celebrate if food didn't exist? What brings you genuine joy?
- Control eating (managing chaos/powerlessness). Think about: What helps you feel capable? What gives you a sense of order? What makes you feel like you're handling things? What demonstrates your power to yourself?

Exercise 2: Creating Your Emotion-Food Response Plan

When you feel overwhelmed by emotions and food feels like the only solution, having a pre-planned response sequence helps you reclaim choice.
- **Step 1**: Name the feeling, don't try to change it yet. Just identify it accurately: 'I'm feeling anxious about tomorrow's presentation', 'I'm feeling lonely and disconnected.'
- **Step 2**: Acknowledge the food urge: 'I want to eat right now to change how I feel.'
- **Step 3**: Commit to trying one tool from your Emotional Regulation Toolkit for just ten minutes.

HOW DIETS MAKE US FAT

If you still want to eat after ten minutes, you can – often the urgency passes or lessens – either way, you've practised tolerating discomfort.

- **Step 4**: Reclaim your hands If you choose to eat. Acknowledge: 'I am choosing to eat for comfort right now.' No shame – just awareness. This is data, not failure.
- **Step 5**: Review which tools actually help shift your emotional state. Which emotions are hardest to sit with? This isn't about never eating emotionally, it's about having actual choices when emotions spike, rather than food being your only automatic response.

Chapter 26

Step 9 – Real-Life Application

Navigating Complex Scenarios

Real life rarely fits neatly into the categories we've established. You'll face situations that combine multiple challenges: social events when your power is low, travel during emotional difficulties, challenging foods in stressful circumstances, disrupted routines when you're already struggling with other areas of your Flight Record.

This step teaches you how to adapt your framework dynamically, rather than abandoning it when life gets complicated.

Dynamic Adaptation

The key to real-life application is understanding that your framework is designed to be adapted, not followed rigidly.

The tools you've learned are meant to be combined, modified, and scaled based on your circumstances. So you need to become familiar with:
- Using multiple tools simultaneously rather than one at a time
- Scaling your expectations based on your current circumstances
- Making conscious trade-offs rather than trying to be perfect in all areas
- Prioritizing the most important elements when you can't maintain everything
- Returning to your foundation when situations become overwhelming

The goal isn't to maintain your ideal approach in all circumstances – it's to maintain your sense of agency and self-care regardless of what's happening around you.

Social Eating Strategies

Social eating presents unique challenges because it adds external pressure, disrupted routines, and emotional complexity to food decisions. Here's how to handle various social eating scenarios.

Restaurants and Social Meals

Before going out, assess your power and decide how you want to approach the meal. Do you want to stick closely to your Baseline eating, or is this an occasion where you want to be more flexible? Either choice is valid, but making the decision in advance prevents in-the-moment confusion.

If you're choosing flexibility, set boundaries that feel good to you. You might decide to enjoy the meal without restriction but return to Baseline eating the next day. The key is that you're making conscious choices rather than feeling swept along by circumstances. If your power is low and you need to stay close to your Baseline, plan ahead by looking at the menu, deciding what you'll order, and preparing responses to any food noise that comes up.

Parties and Celebrations

Social events with challenging foods require preparation and conscious decision-making. Before attending, decide whether this is a Flight Record opportunity (if your power is high) or a situation where you'd rather stick to safer choices.

If you're working with challenging foods, decide in advance what your boundaries are. You might choose to have one piece of cake, or to focus on savory options, or to eat before you go so you're not hungry at the event. Whatever you choose, make it a conscious decision rather than a reactive one.

Practise responses for when people comment on your food choices or try to pressure you to eat things you'd rather not. Simple phrases like 'I'm good, thank you' or 'That looks delicious, but I'm full' usually suffice. Most people are far less focused on your food choices than you think they are.

Travel and Disrupted Routines

Travel disrupts all your normal systems – meal timing, food availability, sleep schedules, stress levels. The key is adapting your framework rather than abandoning it.

Preparation Strategies

Before travelling, assess which aspects of your Baseline you can maintain and which will need to be modified. If you're going somewhere with limited food options, pack Baseline foods or research restaurants in advance. If your sleep will be disrupted, plan for lower power and adjust your expectations accordingly.

Accept that travel days often require Bridge Day choices that might slow your progress – prioritizing not making things worse over maintaining your usual standards. This isn't failure; it's appropriate adaptation to circumstances.

During Travel

Focus on maintaining the most important elements of your framework: power assessment, basic self-care, and agency reclaiming. Your Baseline might look different, but you can still make conscious choices about food and treat yourself kindly.

Use travel as an opportunity to practise flexibility and trust in yourself. Each time you navigate an unusual food situation successfully, you're building evidence that you can handle variety and unpredictability.

HOW DIETS MAKE US FAT

Returning Home

After travel, resist the urge to immediately restrict or 'make up for' any choices you made while away. Return to your Baseline gradually and focus on getting back into your normal routines without drama or punishment.

If you made choices during travel that don't align with your goals, treat them as information rather than failures. What circumstances led to those choices? What could you do differently next time? What did you learn about yourself?

Chapter 27

Step 10 – Long-Term Maintenance and Your Comprehensive Toolkit

Understanding Maintenance Versus Getting There

Now that you've developed skills for navigating complex real-life situations, we need to address the most crucial aspect of this entire framework: how to maintain your long-term progress. This is where most approaches fail, because they focus exclusively on losing weight without teaching you how to keep it off.

The beautiful paradox of this framework is that you've been practising maintenance all along. Your Baseline was designed from day one as a maintenance approach – how you'll eat to keep weight off, not how you'll eat to lose it. Every tool you've learned has been designed for sustainability rather than short-term results.

But maintenance isn't just about continuing to do the

same things forever. It's about understanding how your relationship with food will continue to evolve, how to handle new challenges as they arise, and how to keep building evidence of your capability throughout your life.

What Maintenance Looks Like

Maintenance doesn't look like perfect adherence to your original Baseline plan. It looks like having developed enough skills and self-trust that you can navigate any food situation with confidence:

- Making food decisions based on what serves your current circumstances rather than rigid rules
- Handling disruptions to your routine without panic or complete derailment
- Adapting your approach as your life changes without losing your foundation
- Using challenging food situations as opportunities to build further evidence rather than threats to avoid
- Trusting yourself to handle whatever comes up, even if it's something you haven't encountered before

Maintenance doesn't look like:
- Never making choices you regret
- Never using Bridge Days
- Having the same eating patterns you had during your initial learning period
- Being immune to stress, emotions, or life circumstances affecting your eating

- Never experiencing food noise

The goal of maintenance is not perfection – it's unshakeable self-trust around food.

How Your Framework Evolves Over Time

As you develop mastery with your framework, it will naturally evolve and become more sophisticated:

- **Early Implementation**: During this period, you're actively learning each tool and building basic evidence of your capability. You're following your power assessment religiously, referring to your Baseline plan frequently, and consciously applying your various tools. This feels effortful but manageable.
- **Developing Confidence**: The tools start feeling more natural, and you begin adapting them instinctively to different situations. Your power assessment becomes automatic, your Baseline feels increasingly natural, and you trust yourself to handle more challenging situations.
- **Integration**: Your framework becomes largely invisible – you're using the tools without consciously thinking about them. Food decisions feel neutral most of the time, and you handle challenging situations with confidence. You've built substantial evidence of your capability.
- **Mastery**: You've developed intuitive expertise about what serves you and what doesn't. You can adapt to

any situation while maintaining your sense of self-care. Food is truly neutral – a source of nourishment and pleasure rather than stress or drama.

Common Maintenance Challenges

Even with a solid framework, you'll encounter predictable challenges during maintenance. Understanding these helps you prepare for them rather than being derailed by them:

When the Honeymoon Period Ends

Initially, everything feels new and exciting. You're motivated by progress and the relief of finally having tools that work. Eventually, this novelty wears off, and maintaining your approach can start feeling routine or even boring. This is normal and not a sign that the framework isn't working anymore. It's actually a sign that your new relationship with food is becoming normal rather than something special you have to maintain.

The Urge to 'Level Up' or Restrict

Sometimes, especially during periods when your weight fluctuates upwards or you feel like you're not 'doing enough', you may feel tempted to add further restriction or 'tighten up' your approach. Resist this urge. Weight fluctuations are normal, and adding restriction will likely trigger the old restrict-binge cycle that got you into trouble in the first place. Instead, return to your foundational tools and trust the process.

Comparison and Perfectionism

You might find yourself comparing your maintenance approach to others' dieting efforts, especially when friends are losing weight quickly on new restrictive approaches. Remember that you're playing a different game – you're building skills for life rather than pursuing short-term results. You might also find yourself wanting to perfect your approach or eliminate all challenging eating experiences. This perfectionism can actually undermine your maintenance by making you afraid of normal human imperfection.

Building Your Personal Expertise

One of the most important aspects of long-term maintenance is developing expertise about your own patterns, needs, and responses. Over time, you become the world's leading expert on your own relationship with food.

Recognizing Your Patterns

After using your framework for an extended period, you'll start recognizing subtle patterns that weren't visible initially:
- Which life circumstances consistently affect your power
- How different emotions show up in your eating patterns
- Which foods or eating contexts require more bandwidth

- What early warning signs indicate you need extra support
- Which tools work best for you in different situations

Trusting Your Intuition

As you build evidence of your capability, you'll develop intuitive knowledge about what serves you. This intuition becomes more reliable than external rules or advice because it's based on your actual lived experience.

Learn to distinguish between intuition based on evidence and impulses based on old patterns. Intuition feels calm and grounded; impulses feel urgent and emotionally charged.

Adapting Versus Starting Over

When your current approach isn't working well, resist the urge to throw everything out and start over with a new system. Instead, adapt your existing framework to better serve your current circumstances. Most problems can be solved by returning to basics rather than adding complexity. If your eating feels chaotic, the solution, as you know, is a more consistent power assessment and Baseline practices, not extremes.

The Evolution of Your Process

As you maintain your framework over time, your identity around food gradually shifts from someone who struggles with eating to someone who has a calm, confident relationship with food.

From Chronic Dieter to Someone Who Takes Care of Themselves

Initially, you might still think of yourself as someone who has problems with food but is managing them well. Gradually, this shifts to simply being someone who takes care of themselves around food.

Eventually, you may not think about your relationship with food at all – it just becomes part of how you take care of yourself, like brushing your teeth or getting enough sleep.

From External Rules to Internal Wisdom

Your focus shifts from following external guidelines to trusting your own developed wisdom about what serves you. You become less interested in what diet culture says you should do and more interested in what your own experience has taught you.

From Problem-Focused to Growth-Focused

Instead of trying to fix problems with your eating, you focus on continuing to develop your capabilities. Food situations become opportunities to practise skills rather than dangers to avoid.

Celebrating Subtle Victories

Maintenance victories are often subtle and easy to overlook:
- Handling a stressful period and realizing later there was no food noise during it

- Enjoying a celebration meal, really tasting everything and not feeling any guilt
- Adapting to an unforeseen need for routine change and feeling clear about what to expect and how to go about it
- Then, as you maintain your framework over time, you may notice its effects extending beyond just your relationship with food

Looking Ahead

Maintenance is about maintaining the same core principles – self-compassion, evidence-based decision making, trust in your own wisdom, and commitment to your wellbeing – while allowing your specific practices to evolve as your life changes.

The framework you've learned is designed to grow with you. The power assessment you do at different life stages might look different, but the principle of tuning into your actual capacity remains the same. Your Baseline might evolve as your preferences and circumstances change, but the commitment to eating in a way that feels both nourishing and sustainable remains constant.

What doesn't change:
- Your commitment to treating yourself with kindness
- Your trust in evidence over emotion when making decisions
- Your understanding that perfection isn't required for success

- Your knowledge that you can handle whatever comes up

What continues to evolve:
- Your specific eating preferences and patterns
- Your understanding of what circumstances affect your power
- Your skill level at handling challenging situations
- Your confidence in your own wisdom

The ultimate goal of this entire framework has never been to control your eating perfectly or to eliminate all food challenges from your life. The goal has been to develop unshakeable trust in your ability to take care of yourself around food, regardless of what life brings.

You are not the same person who started this book. You've developed skills, gathered evidence, and built a foundation that will serve you for the rest of your life. The framework becomes part of who you are rather than something you have to remember to do.

Your relationship with food can now be what it was always meant to be: a source of nourishment and pleasure rather than stress and struggle. You've reclaimed your hands, your agency, and your trust in yourself. You've learned that you were never broken – you just needed the right tools and enough evidence to remember what you were always capable of.

This is not the end of your journey – it's the beginning of the rest of your life with food freedom.

Your New Beginning

If you've worked through this framework thoroughly, you've:

- **Understood the true problem**: You've learned that food noise, not willpower, is what's been driving your struggles. You've seen how diet culture has systematically created the problems it claims to solve.
- **Developed a comprehensive assessment system**: You can now evaluate your daily capacity and choose appropriate approaches based on your actual bandwidth rather than wishful thinking.
- **Built a sustainable foundation**: Your Baseline gives you a home base that feels good to return to, rather than a prison you're trying to escape.
- **Created a crisis management system**: Your Bridge Days mean you never have to start from zero again, no matter how difficult things get.
- **Learned to build evidence systematically**: Your Flight Record transforms abstract goals into concrete skills that get easier with practise.
- **Reclaimed your agency**: You understand that you're always in control, even when making choices you regret.
- **Developed strategies for challenging foods**: You can now include or exclude foods based on what serves you, not what diet culture says you should do.
- **Learned to adjust your internal voice**: You've learned how to speak to yourself like someone who believes in your capability rather than someone looking for evidence of your failure.

- **Built emotional regulation skills**: You have tools to process difficult feelings without automatically reaching for food.
- **Seen the real-life application**: You can adapt your framework to any situation rather than abandoning it when life gets complicated.

Most importantly, I hope you're now convinced that you can trust yourself around food. And this faith in your ability to make the next best choice, to take advice from the calmest, wisest version of yourself, will continue growing stronger with each choice you make from a place of self-care rather than self-control.

The Eagle Remembers How to Fly

You've spent this entire journey remembering what you always were. You were never someone who needed to be controlled and restricted. You were always someone who simply needed to remember your true nature and develop the skills to stay in the sky.

The glimpses of food freedom you've had throughout your life weren't flukes or temporary permissions – they were moments when you briefly remembered who you really are. This framework has taught you how to live in that space consistently.

You now know how to:
- Navigate storms without crashing to the ground
- Find nourishment when you need it

- Rest when you're tired without guilt
- Soar when conditions are right
- Trust your wings to carry you

The pen you lived in for so long wasn't your natural habitat – it was a construct created by diet culture to keep you trapped and keep you buying solutions to problems they created. You've broken free not through force or restriction, but by developing the skills that were always yours.

This Time Is Different

You haven't just learned what to do – you've learned why you do it and how to adapt when circumstances change. You haven't just followed another plan – you've developed wisdom about your own patterns and needs.

This time is different because you've addressed the root cause – food noise and the shame spiral it creates – rather than just the symptoms. You've learned to create the same conditions that appetite suppressants provide, but through developing your own skills rather than external intervention.

This time is different because you've built something sustainable. Your framework is designed to grow with you, rather than being something you eventually outgrow or rebel against.

Most importantly, this time is different because you've changed your relationship with struggle itself. Instead of seeing difficulties as evidence that you're failing, you understand them as opportunities to build further evidence of your capability.

What to Expect Moving Forward

Your relationship with food will continue evolving for the rest of your life, but now you have the tools to navigate that evolution with confidence rather than fear.

You'll still have moments of challenge – times when your power is low, when emotions run high, when circumstances disrupt your routines. But these moments will feel different now. Instead of signalling that you're broken or failing, they'll be opportunities to practise your skills and build further evidence.

You'll notice that food noise becomes increasingly impersonal and irrelevant. It doesn't disappear entirely, but it stops controlling your choices. It becomes background static rather than urgent commands.

You'll find that your confidence generalizes beyond food. The self-trust and evidence-building approach you've learned will serve you in every area where you want sustainable change.

Final Reminders

Here are some reminders about the actions that will help you in the future:

- **Continuing to gather evidence**: Every food choice is an opportunity to build further proof of your capability. Don't dismiss successes as flukes or minimize your progress.
- **Adapting your tools**: As your life changes, adapt

your framework rather than abandoning it. The principles remain constant even when the specific applications evolve.
- **Practicing self-compassion**: Be as kind to yourself as you would be to someone you love who is learning something difficult. Perfection is never the goal.
- **Maintaining perspective**: Remember that individual food choices matter less than the overall pattern of treating yourself with care and respect.

This framework is comprehensive, but it's also just the beginning. You now have a foundation for lifelong learning about yourself and your relationship with food.

Stay curious about:
- How your needs evolve as your life changes
- What new evidence you can gather about your capability
- How you can continue simplifying and strengthening your approach
- What other areas of your life could benefit from these same principles

And, as you move forward, remember:
- You were never broken. You were struggling with an impossible task designed to make you fail. Your struggles were evidence of your sanity, not your weakness.
- Food is fuel and pleasure, not moral judgment or

emotional management. The drama around food was learned and can be unlearned.
- You can trust yourself. You've gathered extensive evidence of your capability. Trust that evidence over old fears and doubts.
- Progress isn't linear. Expect ups and downs, and remember that both are part of the learning process.
- You have everything you need. The tools you've learned are comprehensive and will serve you for life. You don't need to keep searching for the next solution.
- This is your new beginning. Not just with food, but with trusting yourself, treating yourself with kindness, and building the life you actually want.

For a minute there, you just forgot you can do whatever you like.

References

American Psychiatric Association. (2013). *Diagnostic and statistical manual of mental disorders* (5th ed.). American Psychiatric Publishing.

Avena, N. M., Rada, P., & Hoebel, B. G. (2008). Evidence for sugar addiction: Behavioral and neurochemical effects of intermittent, excessive sugar intake. *Neuroscience & Biobehavioral Reviews, 32*(1), 20–39.

Bacon, L., & Aphramor, L. (2011). Weight science: Evaluating the evidence for a paradigm shift. *Nutrition Journal, 10,* 9.

Biederman, J., Ball, S. W., Monuteaux, M. C., Surman, C. B., Johnson, J. L., & Zeitlin, S. (2007). Are girls with ADHD at risk for eating disorders? Results from a controlled, five-year prospective study. *Journal of Developmental & Behavioral Pediatrics, 28*(4), 302–307.

Brockmeyer, T., Skunde, M., Wu, M., Bresslein, E., Rudofsky, G., Herzog, W., & Friederich, H. C. (2014). Difficulties in emotion regulation across the spectrum of eating disorders. *Comprehensive Psychiatry, 55*(3), 565–571.

Brownell, K. D., & Rodin, J. (1994). Medical, metabolic, and psychological effects of weight cycling. *Archives of Internal Medicine, 154*(12), 1325–1330.

Cortese, S., Angriman, M., Maffeis, C., Isnard, P., Konofal, E., Lecendreux, M., Purper-Ouakil, D., Vincenzi, B., Bernardina, B. D., & Mouren, M. C. (2008). Attention-deficit/hyperactivity disorder (ADHD) and obesity: A systematic review of the literature. *Critical Reviews in Food Science and Nutrition, 48*(6), 524–537.

Dearing, R. L., Stuewig, J., & Tangney, J. P. (2005). On the importance of distinguishing shame from guilt: Relations to problematic alcohol and drug use. *Addictive Behaviors, 30*(7), 1392–1404.

Dickerson, S. S., Gruenewald, T. L., & Kemeny, M. E. (2004). When the social self is threatened: Shame, physiology, and health. *Journal of Personality, 72*(6), 1191–1216.

Docet, M. F., Lasat, S., Brogna, P., Mazza, M., Marano, G., Muti-Schumaker, P., & Janiri, L. (2012). Adult ADHD and comorbid eating disorders in an Italian adult ADHD population. *Journal of Psychopathology, 18,* 130–136.

Dulloo, A. G., & Montani, J. P. (2015). Pathways from dieting to weight regain, to obesity and to the metabolic syndrome: An overview. *Obesity Reviews, 16*(S1), 1–6.

Eisenberger, N. I., Lieberman, M. D., & Williams, K. D. (2003). Does rejection hurt? An fMRI study of social pain. *Science, 302*(5643), 290–292.

Evans, J. St. B. T., & Stanovich, K. E. (2013). Dual-process theories of higher cognition: Advancing the debate. *Perspectives on Psychological Science, 8*(3), 223–241.

Fazzino, T. L., Rohde, K., & Sullivan, D. K. (2019). Hyper-palatable foods: Development of a quantitative definition and application to the US food system database. *Obesity, 27*(11), 1761–1768.

Felitti, V. J., Anda, R. F., Nordenberg, D., Williamson, D. F., Spitz, A. M., Edwards, V., Koss, M. P., & Marks, J. S. (1998). Relationship of childhood abuse and household dysfunction to many of the leading causes of death in adults. *American Journal of Preventive Medicine, 14*(4), 245–258.

Field, A. E., Austin, S. B., Taylor, C. B., Malspeis, S., Rosner, B., Rockett, H. R., Gillman, M. W., & Colditz, G. A. (2003). Relation between dieting and weight change among preadolescents and adolescents. *Pediatrics, 112*(4), 900–906.

Fothergill, E., Guo, J., Howard, L., Kerns, J. C., Knuth, N. D., Brychta, R., Chen, K. Y., Skarulis, M. C., Walter, M., Walter, P. J., & Hall, K. D. (2016). Persistent metabolic adaptation 6 years after "The Biggest Loser" competition. *Obesity, 24*(8), 1612–1619.

Gearhardt, A. N., Corbin, W. R., & Brownell, K. D. (2009). Preliminary validation of the Yale Food Addiction Scale. *Appetite, 52*(2), 430–436.

Gearhardt, A. N., Yokum, S., Orr, P. T., Stice, E., Corbin, W. R., & Brownell, K. D. (2011). Neural correlates of food addiction. *Archives of General Psychiatry, 68*(8), 808–816.

Gilbert, P., & Irons, C. (2005). Focused therapies and compassionate mind training for shame and self-attacking. In P. Gilbert (Ed.), *Compassion: Conceptualisations, research and use in psychotherapy* (pp. 325–263). Routledge.

Grabe, S., Ward, L. M., & Hyde, J. S. (2008). The role of the media in body image concerns among women: A meta-analysis of experimental and correlational studies. *Psychological Bulletin, 134*(3), 460–476.

Haedt-Matt, A. A., & Keel, P. K. (2011). Revisiting the affect regulation model of binge eating: A meta-analysis of studies using ecological momentary assessment. *Psychological Bulletin, 137*(4), 660–681.

Hall, K. D., Ayuketah, A., Brychta, R., Cai, H., Cassimatis, T., Chen, K. Y., Chung, S. T., Costa, E., Courville, A., Darcey, V., Fletcher, L. A., Forde, C. G., Gharib, A. M., Guo, J., Howard, R., Joseph, P. V., McGehee, S., Ouwerkerk, R., Raisinger, K., ... Zhou, M. (2019). Ultra-processed diets cause excess calorie intake and weight gain: An inpatient randomized controlled trial of ad libitum food intake. *Cell Metabolism, 30*(1), 67 77.e3.

Harrison, K. (2000). The body electric: Thin-ideal media and eating disorders in adolescents. *Journal of Communication, 50*(3), 119–143.

Herbert, B. M., & Pollatos, O. (2014). Attenuated interoceptive sensitivity in overweight and obese individuals. *Eating Behaviors, 15*(3), 445–448.

Herman, C. P., & Polivy, J. (1980). Restrained eating. In A. J. Stunkard (Ed.), *Obesity* (pp. 225–208). W. B. Saunders.

Herman, C. P., & Polivy, J. (1984). A boundary model for the regulation of eating. *Research Publications – Association for Research in Nervous and Mental Disease, 62*, 141–156.

Jackson, S. E., Beeken, R. J., & Wardle, J. (2014). Perceived weight discrimination and changes in weight, waist circumference, and weight status. *Obesity, 22*(12), 2485–2488.

Jenkinson, P. M., Taylor, L., & Laws, K. R. (2018). Self-reported interoceptive deficits in eating disorders: A meta-analysis of studies using the eating disorder inventory. *Journal of Psychosomatic Research, 110*, 38–45.

Kahneman, D. (2011). *Thinking, fast and slow*. Farrar, Straus and Giroux.

Kaisari, P., Dourish, C. T., & Higgs, S. (2017). Attention deficit hyperactivity disorder (ADHD) and disordered eating behaviour: A systematic review and a framework for future research. *Clinical Psychology Review, 53*, 109–121.

Kelly, N. R., Bulik, C. M., & Mazzeo, S. E. (2013). Executive functioning and behavioral impulsivity of young women who binge eat. *International Journal of Eating Disorders*, 46(2), 127–135.

Khalsa, S. S., Adolphs, R., Cameron, O. G., Critchley, H. D., Davenport, P. W., Feinstein, J. S., Feusner, J. D., Garfinkel, S. N., Lane, R. D., Mehling, W. E., Meuret, A. E., Nemeroff, C. B., Oppenheimer, S., Petzschner, F. H., Pollatos, O., Rhudy, J. L., Schramm, L. P., Simmons, W. K., Stein, M. B., ... Paulus, M. P. (2018). Interoception and mental health: A roadmap. *Biological Psychiatry: Cognitive Neuroscience and Neuroimaging*, 3(6), 501–513.

Larimer, M. E., Palmer, R. S., & Marlatt, G. A. (1999). Relapse prevention: An overview of Marlatt's cognitive-behavioral model. *Alcohol Research & Health*, 23(2), 151–160.

Leehr, E. J., Krohmer, K., Schag, K., Dresler, T., Zipfel, S., & Giel, K. E. (2015). Emotion regulation model in binge eating disorder and obesity – A systematic review. *Neuroscience & Biobehavioral Reviews*, 49, 125–134.

Lichtman, S. W., Pisarska, K., Berman, E. R., Pestone, M., Dowling, H., Offenbacher, E., Weisel, H., Heshka, S., Matthews, D. E., & Heymsfield, S. B. (1992). Discrepancy between self-reported and actual caloric intake and exercise in obese subjects. *New England Journal of Medicine*, 327(27), 1893–1898.

Lowe, M. R., & Levine, A. S. (2005). Eating motives and the controversy over dieting: Eating less than needed versus less than wanted. *Obesity Research*, 13(5), 797–806.

Lowe, M. R., Doshi, S. D., Katterman, S. N., & Feig, E. H. (2013). Dieting and restrained eating as prospective predictors of weight gain. *Frontiers in Psychology*, 4, 577.

Macht, M. (2008). How emotions affect eating: A five-way model. *Appetite*, 50(1), 1–11.

Mann, T., Tomiyama, A. J., Westling, E., Lew, A. M., Samuels, B., & Chatman, J. (2007). Medicare's search for effective obesity treatments: Diets are not the answer. *American Psychologist*, 62(3), 220–233.

Marlatt, G. A. (1996). Harm reduction: Come as you are. *Addictive Behaviors*, 21(6), 779–788.

Marlatt, G. A., & Donovan, D. M. (Eds.). (2005). *Relapse prevention: Maintenance strategies in the treatment of addictive behaviors* (2nd ed.). Guilford Press.

Miller, W. R., & Rollnick, S. (2012). *Motivational interviewing: Helping people change* (3rd ed.). Guilford Press.

Montani, J. P., Schutz, Y., & Dulloo, A. G. (2015). Dieting and weight cycling as risk factors for cardiometabolic diseases: Who is really at risk? *Obesity Reviews*, 16(S1), 7–18.

Nazar, B. P., Bernardes, C., Peachey, G., Sergeant, J., Mattos, P., & Treasure, J. (2016). The risk of eating disorders comorbid with attention-deficit/hyperactivity disorder: A systematic review and meta-analysis. *International Journal of Eating Disorders*, 49(12), 1045–1057.

Neff, K. D. (2003). Self-compassion: An alternative conceptualization of a healthy attitude toward oneself. *Self and Identity*, 2(2), 85–101.

Neumark-Sztainer, D., Wall, M., Story, M., & Standish, A. R. (2012). Dieting and unhealthy weight control behaviors during adolescence: Associations with 10-year changes in body mass index. *Journal of Adolescent Health*, 50(1), 80–86.

Pietiläinen, K. H., Saarni, S. E., Kaprio, J., & Rissanen, A. (2012). Does dieting make you fat? A twin study. *International Journal of Obesity*, 36(3), 456–464.

Polivy, J., & Herman, C. P. (1985). Dieting and binging: A causal analysis. *American Psychologist*, 40(2), 193–201.

Polivy, J., & Herman, C. P. (1999). Distress and eating: Why do dieters overeat? *International Journal of Eating Disorders*, 26(2), 153–164.

Prochaska, J. O., DiClemente, C. C., & Norcross, J. C. (1992). In search of how people change: Applications to addictive behaviors. *American Psychologist*, 47(9), 1102–1114.

Puhl, R. M., & Heuer, C. A. (2009). The stigma of obesity: A review and update. *Obesity*, 17(5), 941–964.

Reinblatt, S. P., Leoutsakos, J. M., Mahone, E. M., Forrester, S., Wilcox, H. C., & Riddle, M. A. (2015). Association between binge eating and attention-deficit/hyperactivity disorder in two pediatric community mental health clinics. *International Journal of Eating Disorders*, 48(5), 505–511.

Richard, A., Meule, A., Reichenberger, J., & Blechert, J. (2017). Food cravings in everyday life: An EMA study on snack-related thoughts, cravings, and consumption. *Appetite*, 113, 215–223.

Rosenbaum, M., & Leibel, R. L. (2010). Adaptive thermogenesis in humans. *International Journal of Obesity*, 34(Suppl. 1), S47–S55.

Schaefer, J. T., & Magnuson, A. B. (2014). A review of interventions that promote eating by internal cues. *Journal of the Academy of Nutrition and Dietetics*, 114(5), 734–760.

Schaumberg, K., Anderson, D. A., Anderson, L. M., Reilly, E. E., & Gorrell, S. (2016). Dietary restraint: What's the harm? A review of the relationship between dietary restraint, weight trajectory and the development of eating pathology. *Clinical Obesity*, 6(2), 89–100.

Schoeller, D. A. (1995). Limitations in the assessment of dietary energy intake by self-report. *Metabolism*, 44(2 Suppl 2), 18–22.

Schulte, E. M., Avena, N. M., & Gearhardt, A. N. (2015). Which foods may be addictive? The roles of processing, fat content, and glycemic load. *PLOS ONE*, 10(2), e0117959.

Seitz, J., Kahraman-Lanzerath, B., Legenbauer, T., Sarrar, L., Herpertz, S., Salbach-Andrae, H., Konrad, K., & Herpertz-Dahlmann, B. (2013). The role of impulsivity, inattention and comorbid ADHD in patients with bulimia nervosa. *PLOS ONE*, 8(5), e63891.

Small, D. M., & DiFeliceantonio, A. G. (2019). Processed foods and food reward. *Science*, 363(6425), 346–347.

Sonneville, K. R., Calzo, J. P., Horton, N. J., Field, A. E., Crosby, R. D., Solmi, F., & Micali, N. (2015). Childhood hyperactivity/inattention and eating disturbances predict binge eating in adolescence. *Psychological Medicine*, 45(12), 2511–2520.

Stevenson, R. J., Francis, H. M., Attuquayefio, T., Gupta, D., Yeomans, M. R., Oaten, M. J., & Davidson, T. (2020). Hippocampal-dependent appetitive control is impaired by experimental exposure to a Western-style diet. *Royal Society Open Science*, 7(2), 191338.

Stice, E., Presnell, K., & Spangler, D. (2002). Risk factors for binge eating onset in adolescent girls: A 2-year prospective investigation. *Health Psychology*, 21(2), 131–138.

Stice, E., Sysko, R., Roberto, C. A., & Allison, S. (2010). Are dietary restraint scales valid measures of dietary restriction? Additional objective behavioral and biological data suggest not. *Appetite*, 54(2), 331–339.

Strimas, R., Davis, C., Patte, K., Curtis, C., Reid, C., & McCool, C. (2008). Symptoms of attention-deficit/hyperactivity disorder, overeating, and body mass index in men. *Eating Behaviors*, 9(4), 516–518.

Sumithran, P., Prendergast, L. A., Delbridge, E., Purcell, K., Shulkes, A., Kriketos, A., & Proietto, J. (2011). Long-term persistence of hormonal adaptations to weight loss. *New England Journal of Medicine*, 365(17), 1597–1604.

Sutin, A. R., & Terracciano, A. (2013). Perceived weight discrimination and obesity. *PLOS ONE*, 8(7), e70048.

Tangney, J. P., Stuewig, J., & Mashek, D. J. (2007). Moral emotions and moral behavior. *Annual Review of Psychology*, 58, 345–372.

Tatarsky, A., & Kellogg, S. (2010). Integrative harm reduction psychotherapy: A case of substance use, multiple trauma, and suicidality. *Journal of Clinical Psychology*, 66(2), 123–135.

Thomas, J. J., Vartanian, L. R., & Brownell, K. D. (2009). The relationship between eating disorder not otherwise specified (EDNOS) and officially recognized eating disorders: Meta-analysis and implications for DSM. *Psychological Bulletin*, 135(3), 407–433.

Tomiyama, A. J. (2014). Weight stigma is stressful: A review of evidence for the Cyclic Obesity/Weight-Based Stigma model. *Appetite*, 82, 8–15.

Tomiyama, A. J., Carr, D., Granberg, E. M., Major, B., Robinson, E., Sutin, A. R., & Brewis, A. (2018). How and why weight stigma drives the obesity 'epidemic' and harms health. *BMC Medicine*, 16, 123.

Urbszat, D., Herman, C. P., & Polivy, J. (2002). Eat, drink, and be merry, for tomorrow we diet: Effects of anticipated deprivation on food intake in restrained and unrestrained eaters. *Journal of Abnormal Psychology*, 111(2), 396–401.

Van Dyke, N., & Drinkwater, E. J. (2014). Relationships between intuitive eating and health indicators: Literature review. *Public Health Nutrition*, 17(8), 1757–1766.

van Strien, T., & Ouwens, M. A. (2007). Effects of distress, alexithymia and impulsivity on eating. *Eating Behaviors*, 8(2), 251–257.

Volkow, N. D., & Morales, M. (2015). The brain on drugs: From reward to addiction. *Cell*, 162(4), 712–725.

Westenhoefer, J., Stunkard, A. J., & Pudel, V. (1999). Validation of the flexible and rigid control dimensions of dietary restraint. *International Journal of Eating Disorders*, 26(1), 53–64.

Witkiewitz, K., & Marlatt, G. A. (2004). Relapse prevention for alcohol and drug problems: That was Zen, this is Tao. *American Psychologist*, 59(4), 224–235.

Wong, M., & Qian, M. (2016). The role of shame in emotional eating. *Appetite*, 106, 29–35.